HELP
Your Man
GET HEALTHY

HELP
Your Man
GET HEALTHY

AN ESSENTIAL GUIDE
FOR EVERY CARING WOMAN

MARIA KASSBERG REGAN
AND STEVEN JONAS, M.D.

AN AVON BOOK

The information in this book is not intended to serve as a replacement for medical care. It is strongly advised that you consult a physician before acting on any information herein.

AVON BOOKS, INC.
1350 Avenue of the Americas
New York, New York 10019

Copyright © 1999 by Maria Kassberg and Steven M. Jonas, M.D.
Interior design by Rhea Braunstein
Published by arrangement with the authors
ISBN: 0-380-79769-0
www.avonbooks.com/wholecare

Library of Congress Cataloging in Publication Data:

Regan, Maria Kassberg.
    Help your man get healthy : an essential guide for every caring woman / Maria Kassberg Regan, Steven Jonas.
        p.   cm.
    "An Avon book."
    1. Men—Health and hygiene. I. Jonas, Steven. II. Title.
RA777.8.R445   1999   99-25808
613'.04234—dc21   CIP

First WholeCare Printing: June 1999

WHOLECARE TRADEMARK REG. U.S. PAT. OFF. AND IN OTHER COUNTRIES, MARCA REGISTRADA, HECHO EN U.S.A.

Printed in the U.S.A.

OPM   10 9 8 7 6 5 4 3 2 1

CONTENTS

INTRODUCTION:
WHY SHOULD YOU HELP
YOUR MAN GET HEALTHY?

There is no way to make people like change. You can only make them feel less threatened by it.

Frederick O R. Hayes

How long can you expect to live? Will it be 95 years or 45 years? Believe it or not, you can estimate the length of your life—and that of your partner—on the Internet, among other places. The longevity game at Northwestern Mutual Life Insurance Company's Web site gives the bottom line on unhealthy habits (see pages 3–4).

Here are some examples: smokers who go through two or more packs of cigarettes a day can expect to live an average of eight years fewer than if they didn't smoke. People who have been convicted of driving while intoxicated can expect to live about six years fewer than they would have otherwise. A simple thing like not knowing what your blood pressure is reduces life expectancy by two years. On the other hand, maintaining a healthy weight adds about two years to your life, and always wearing a seat belt in the car adds about one.

Medical research confirms insurance industry experience. Studies have shown conclusively that both heart disease and cancer—the top two killers in the nation—can be prevented by avoiding certain negative health habits and engaging in certain positive ones. We're so used to thinking of ourselves as victims of disease that it's not easy to comprehend that, in many cases, we're our own assailants.

According to the National Institutes of Health, lifestyle changes can reduce heart disease risk as follows: within five years of quitting, a former smoker is 50 to 70 percent less likely to have a heart attack than a current smoker. A person who exercises regularly is 45 percent less likely to have a heart attack than a person who is sedentary. A person who maintains a healthy weight is 35 to 55 percent less likely to have a heart attack than someone who is 20 percent or more overweight.

As for cancer risk, a 1996 study from the Harvard School of Public Health found that an astonishing 65 percent of cancer deaths could be prevented by lifestyle changes. The Harvard researchers found that 30 percent of cancer deaths are due to smoking, 30 percent to poor diet and obesity, and 5 percent to lack of exercise.

The bottom line, according to former acting Surgeon General Audrey Manley, M.D., is that about half of all deaths that occur in the United States each year have their roots in personal behavior. Of course, even people who exercise, eat right, and don't smoke die of heart disease and cancer. But at any given age, considerably fewer of them die than do people who are more careless with their health (the sedentary, the overweight, and the smokers). For many, healthy habits mark the difference between a life that's long and vigorous and one that's curtailed by chronic disease or shortened by death.

HOW UNHEALTHY HABITS CAN CUT LIFE SHORT

Northwestern Mutual Life Insurance Company has devised a "Longevity Game" that you can play at its Web site (northwesternmutual. com/games/longevity/). In the game, various habits are assigned a score (plus or minus a certain number of years of life expectancy) based on insurance industry research. Here's a sampling of what some habits can do to the length of a life:

Bad Habit	Average Number of Years Lost	Good Habit	Average Number of Years Gained
Smoking (more than two packs a day)	−8	Never having smoked	+2
Having been convicted of driving while intoxicated (in the last five years)	−6	No moving violations (in the last year)	+1
Having 5 or more drinks one or more times per week	−6	Never drinking more than three drinks in a day	+1
Smoking (less than two packs a day)	−4	—	
Being overweight	−4	Maintaining a healthy weight	+2

Bad Habit	Average Number of Years Lost	Good Habit	Average Number of Years Gained
Being inactive	−3	Exercising regularly	+3
Drinking three or four drinks (three or more times a week)	−3	——	
Eating saturated fat indiscriminately	−2	Eating saturated fat sparingly	+2
Not managing stress	−1	Managing stress well	+1

One Man's Wake-Up Call

"My husband never would have quit smoking if he hadn't had a heart attack," says Ava Meade. The first occured one month before Bob turned 34 years old. Fortunately, Bob's heart wasn't damaged. He had been given a warning—an opportunity to stave off a second, more damaging attack. Although he made some dietary changes, he continued to smoke cigarettes away from home.

About a year later, Bob had a second heart attack which killed 5 percent of his heart muscle.

It has been three years since the second heart attack. Bob and Ava walk two miles five times a week. Bob no longer smokes—anywhere. The couple met with a nutritionist to learn which foods Bob should avoid and which he should eat more of. Now when Ava's grocery shopping, the breakfast foods she selects include Cheerios and oatmeal cereal rather than bacon and eggs, which Bob used to have for breakfast every day. When Ava buys meat, she selects a low-fat cut, which she'll grill rather than fry.

Why should a woman take on the task of helping her partner overhaul his lifestyle? "You need two people to do this," says Ava. "There's a lot to remember. And you need someone to support you—a buddy. The best person for that is your spouse."

The effort of changing the family diet and accompanying Bob on his walks has paid off for Ava in many ways. She herself has a family history of high cholesterol and heart disease, so she's protecting her own health—and that of the couple's two daughters—while helping her spouse protect his. And there's another benefit. "Now," says Ava, "I can sleep with him without wondering if he's going to drop dead next to me."

Make no mistake, helping your partner change unhealthy habits could save his life. Undeniably, having a heart attack—or two—is a motivating force that's hard to match. But *Help Your Man Get Healthy* will show you many other ways to help the man in your life mobilize his motivation, get healthier, and stay on that road for the rest of his life.

FOUR STEPS TO A HEALTHIER LIFE

In 1997, the American Heart Association issued simplified recommendations for preventing heart disease through diet and other lifestyle issues such as smoking and weight management. The American Cancer Society updated its guidelines for diet, nutrition, and cancer prevention in 1996. The following is a combination of both sets of recommendations.

1. Stop smoking. Smoking damages the inner walls of arteries, making them more prone to collect fatty deposits called plaque. Plaque buildup can lead to blockages that keep blood from reaching the heart, which causes a heart attack. If the blockage prevents blood from reaching the brain, it causes a stroke. Smoking also causes cancer and chronic lung diseases, impairs fertility, increases risk of osteoporosis, and significantly adds to the long-term health risks of people who have diabetes.

2. Adopt a healthy diet. Fifty percent of American men will develop cancer in their lifetime. Forty-two percent will develop heart disease. The good news: Both can be prevented through a healthy diet. You can achieve a healthy diet by following these guidelines from the American Cancer Society:

A. Choose most of the foods you eat from plant sources.
  - Eat five or more servings of fruits and vegetables each day.
  - Eat other foods from plant sources, such as breads, cereals, grain products, rice, pasta, or beans several times each day.
B. Limit your intake of high-fat foods, particularly from animal sources.
  - Choose foods low in fat.
  - Limit consumption of meats, especially high-fat meats.
C. Limit consumption of alcoholic beverages, if you drink at all.

3. Maintain a healthy weight. Excess weight increases risk of heart disease, some cancers (including those of the colon, rectum, prostate, and kidney), diabetes, osteoporosis, and osteoarthritis.

4. Make a commitment to exercise. According to the American Heart Association, as many as 250,000 people in the U.S. die each year due to lack of regular physical activity. Exercise helps people maintain a healthy weight, strengthens the heart, and boosts mood and energy. It helps prevent heart disease, some cancers, diabetes, osteoarthritis, and osteoporosis. In fact, it's so important to your man's health that we've devoted a whole chapter to it (see Chapter 5, "Get Your Man Moving)."

How much exercise is enough? The American Cancer Society and other experts recommend that adults be at least moderately active for 30 minutes or more on most days of the week.

Six Reasons to Get Involved

It's clear that most men could stand to improve their health habits (just take a look at the statistics under number 1, "Men need help," below). What's not so clear is why women should take any responsibility at all for men's health. They're grown ups, right? They're capable of understanding that personal habits can have far-reaching positive and negative health effects. And anyway, women have their plates full already. In many homes, women (whether they work or not) are primarily responsible for everything from raising children to cleaning toilets and a multitude of things in between. Isn't that enough responsibility?

Of course it is. Nevertheless, there are good reasons for a woman to add improving her husband's lifestyle to her list of things to do. Here are six:

1. Men need help. Sixty percent of them don't engage in the minimum recommended amount of physical activity (30 to 45 minutes of brisk walking—or its equivalent—daily), and about 25 percent don't engage in *any* leisure-time physical activity. Thirty-three percent of men are overweight, and 28 percent smoke cigarettes. Twenty-eight percent of those who report significant levels of stress aren't doing anything to reduce or better manage that stress.

In addition, many men don't know enough about health. Women's magazines are plentiful and chock-full of health stories. Most men's magazines are neither of those things. In addition, women see their doctors more often than men, which makes them better informed and more likely to pick up a health problem early, when it's most treatable.

One more way women learn about medical issues is that they share health information among themselves. The average man, on the other hand, is unlikely to tell a male friend that he's concerned about his weak urine stream, is afraid he drinks too much, or wants to lose weight. By not doing so, he's missing out on a potentially valuable pool of knowledge. You can learn a lot from a friend who has experienced a health problem similar to your own.

By learning about men's health issues, you can give your partner the information he needs to make smart choices about his lifestyle.

2. Women need help, too. To be fair, we have to point out that women are not without bad health habits. In fact, women are slightly more likely than men to be overweight, and just as unlikely to get enough exercise. Thirty-four percent of women are overweight, 60 percent don't get enough exercise, and more than 25 percent aren't active at all. Twenty-three percent of women smoke.

All the more reason to help your man get healthy. Any change you help him make is likely to rub off on you. Let's say your partner's cholesterol is high, and you make it your project to reduce saturated fat and cholesterol in the family diet. Your arteries will thank you just as heartily as his.

3. Assuming you want your man around for a long time, his health is your concern. Even though the total numbers aren't high, American men aged 25 to 44 are 59 percent more likely to die before the age of 45 than women in their age group. The statistics improve for men aged 45 to 64—they're only 42 percent more likely to die before the age of 65 than women in their age group. Those staggering differences translate to an average of 6.6 fewer years of life for men. If you want to grow old together, now is the time to do something about it.

4. As long as your partner lives recklessly, you'll worry. "Every time he smokes a cigarette or eats a cookie, it kills *you* inside a little bit," says Ava Meade, whose husband, Bob, had those two heart attacks by the age of 35. "If Bob eats a cookie, I worry about that cookie all day. That's not a way anyone should have to live."

5. Helping your partner improve his health habits will make him a better role model for your children. Children learn with their eyes. If they see you and your partner having fruit on your cereal and grabbing an apple or a yogurt when you're hungry, they'll do the same. If your children see you reaching for chips or cookies between meals, they'll do that, too. According to Susan Kalish, author of *Your Child's Fitness: Practical Advice for Parents,* active fathers are 3.5 times more likely to have active children than sedentary dads. In fact, she says, active parents are the most important factor in determining whether children will be active rather than sedentary.

6. A healthy man is an attractive man. If your partner begins a regular exercise program, loses 20 pounds or quits smoking, he'll feel better about himself—and have more stamina. Among other things, that combination is sure to improve your love life.

"His sex drive is much better," says Michelle Bromley of her fiancé, Roman LePree, who lost 40 pounds in 1995 by overhauling his diet and taking up exercise. "You can be a lot more open with each other—and have a lot more fun—when you both feel good about yourselves."

Can a Woman Help Her Man Get Healthy?

Let's assume you've decided you want to invest some time and energy into helping your man get healthy. Can you really make a difference? Yes. According to the Surgeon General's 1996 report on physical activity and health, "social support from family and friends has been consistently and positively related to regular physical activity."

A Gallup survey done for *American Health* magazine in 1985 found that people use the family as an instrument of self-change. People living with others were somewhat more likely to improve their diets or cut down their drinking, especially if there were children at home. Husbands were twice as likely as single men to quit smoking (22 percent versus 11 percent). They also were more likely to lose weight (42 percent versus 31 percent). These numbers correspond to the fact that single people have a shorter life expectancy than those who have a mate.

When Gallup asked respondents who, if anyone, helped them improve their health habits, more people said they were helped by a spouse, boyfriend, girlfriend or family member than by their physician.

That finding is supported by a 1996 study commissioned by the President's Council on Physical Fitness and Sports and the Sporting Goods Manufacturers Association. Of the 1,000 exercise slackers surveyed, 44 percent said their spouse or significant other was the strongest of all external motivating forces—stronger, even, than the force of a doctor's advice.

Having said that you can help your partner lead a healthier life, it's important to point out that while you can suggest, support, and inspire change, you can't make the change for him. That means trying to alter your partner's diet without his consent—by suddenly refusing to buy or cook beef, for example—won't work. Neither will nagging or laying on guilt trips. A woman who wants to help her man get healthy has to walk the fine line between educating and harassing; supporting and threatening; building self-esteem and tearing it down.

The tips, tactics, and techniques in this book will help you encourage healthy changes in your partner's behavior. As you plan your strategy, it's important to remember the obvious: men, like women, are individuals. What works for one may not work for another. So if one approach doesn't inspire your man to change, try a different one. For example, if suggesting that your partner start running with you doesn't get him to lace up his cross-trainers, don't give up. It may simply be that running doesn't appeal to him. He might be more inspired by the competition of a team sport or by a game that involves a skill he can try to master (like golf or tennis).

Soon you'll build up a stable of the motivating thoughts that work best for your partner. Ava Meade has found that avoiding the need for medication motivates her husband. When he gains a little weight, she simply reminds him that if he doesn't lose it, the doctor will probably have to increase the dose of his cholesterol-lowering medication.

People can change most of their bad habits once they find the motivation to do so. However, it's important to realize that there are men who won't change, no matter what you say or do. These men may have psychological issues that can't be resolved without the help of professional therapists or addiction programs. Or it simply may not be the right time for them to change (see Chapter 1 for more information on the psychology of motivation).

Try to accept whatever changes your partner is willing

to make at this time. If he's not ready to quit smoking, encourage him to use a seat belt every time he gets into a car. Although using a seat belt isn't commonly thought of as a health habit, it is. As pointed out earlier, it can add a year to your life. Remember, successfully changing one habit, no matter how simple, lays the groundwork for future changes by boosting one's confidence that changes indeed can be made.

Change is hard for most of us. That's the bad news. The better news is that you *can* create an environment that will encourage your partner to adopt a healthier lifestyle. The best news of all is that you and your partner will likely live a happier, livelier, and longer life as a result of any healthy habit changes you make.

1

MOBILIZE YOUR MAN'S MOTIVATION

> *You can preach a better sermon with your life than with your lips.*
> *Oliver Goldsmith*

Motivation is a word we toss about quite casually. However, to understand how you can help your man get healthy, you need a clear understanding of the word. Here's our definition: Motivation is the mental process that links a thought or feeling to an action.

It's also important to understand the fact that motivation is not something you can give—or force upon—someone else. It has to come from within the person who's going to do the changing.

How do we get motivation? The answer is that we've already got it. Although it may lie dormant for years, the motivation to improve oneself is part of human nature. Think of motivation as a component of the will to live. When people face a perilous situation, they often remember later how their will to live pushed them to overcome whatever physical obstacles stood between them and safety or recovery. We're all familiar with tales of people who showed strength they never thought they had in the face of life-or-death situations. The motivation that we use to succeed at our jobs or to make lifestyle changes is our will to live expressing itself under less dramatic circumstances.

If we all have motivation, why aren't we all perfect models of healthy behavior? Because motivation can be blocked, immobilized, or submerged by any number of events or circumstances. For example, a person is unlikely to change bad habits when he's depressed. He's also unlikely to commit to lifestyle improvements when he's facing a crisis or when he has too many other commitments. If your partner is working full-time while attending college and you've just had a baby, this probably isn't the time to campaign for major lifestyle changes.

Motivation for healthy change is also hard to mobilize when you just plain enjoy an unhealthy behavior, such as eating lots of fatty food, or when you're just plain addicted to an unhealthy substance, such as nicotine in tobacco.

There are exceptions, of course. A medical crisis often unblocks a man's motivation to protect his health. If a man—or someone close to him—suffers a heart attack, there's a good chance he'll realize that he should take better care of himself.

As you formulate your plan to help your man get healthy, remember that your goal isn't to make your partner change his habits; it's to make him *want* to change his habits.

The Steps Toward Change

You'll be better equipped for this task if you're familiar with the psychology of motivation. When it comes to changing habits, how do people move from thought to action? Psychologists J. Prochaska, C. DiClemente, and J.

Norcross have identified eight stages that people go through on their way to healthier behavior. We provide suggestions on how you can help your man get to—and through—each of them.

Precontemplation

At this stage, the person isn't convinced that he has a behavior that needs changing. He may not be aware of the benefits a change would bring, or he may be discouraged because of past failures. In any case, he doesn't think the benefits of changing outweigh the benefits of not changing.

What you can do If your man is at this stage, he's not ready to change. But that doesn't mean that he won't be ready in six months—or that there's nothing you can do now to help him reach the next stage. If he's not ready to quit smoking, for example, he may be ready to take a smaller step toward better health, such as fastening his seat belt whenever he gets into a car.

Tell him you're concerned about his safety on the road, and use a seat belt yourself whenever you're in a car. Explain that starting off with a smaller, less demanding change will help to prepare him for bigger changes that require a higher degree of sacrifice. The success your partner experiences as he begins habitually to buckle his seat belt will empower him later, when he's ready to tackle his smoking habit.

Contemplation

Now the person starts to realize that his habit or behavior is a problem. He's seriously thinking about doing something positive for his health within the next six months. However, he's still keenly aware of the disadvantages of changing his behavior and thinks that it will be difficult to do so.

What you can do Talk to your man. Try to get him to put into words what he sees as the disadvantages of changing the habit in question. Then try to help him see those disadvantages as minor or, even better, convince him that they're really advantages.

For example, let's say your partner wants to start exercising, but he works long hours and feels that an exercise routine would take more time away from the little he has to spend with you and the children. There are a number of possible solutions you might offer. Can he take a walk during his lunch break or work out at a gym near work? Can he get up 45 minutes early to exercise before work? Can he park his car in the spot farthest from the door to the building where he works, then routinely take the stairs instead of the elevator?

If his schedule won't allow either of the first two options, think of ways the family can exercise together. You might join the YMCA or another family health club. The children can take swimming or gymnastics while you and your partner work out. If you have a child who isn't old enough to take a class by himself, you and your partner can take turns working out and playing with the baby. Some Ys and health clubs offer baby-sitting. Another option is to plan active family outings such as swimming, hiking, skiing, or sledding. Including children in exercise plans has the added benefit of keeping them fit and teaching them good health habits.

Preparation

In this stage, the person has found the thoughts and/or feelings that will activate him, and believes that change is possible. In other words, he has unblocked his motivation. This may happen because of a single learning experience, such as hearing about an old friend who was overweight and out of shape and who died suddenly of a heart attack. Or it may be the result of a less dramatic negative experience that keeps repeating itself, such as getting out of breath every time he climbs a flight of stairs. At this stage, the person is planning to change his problem behavior within the next month.

What you can do Help him find the resources he'll need to make the changes he wants to make. Buy him a subscription to a men's magazine that focuses on health and fitness. If he's going to quit smoking, talk to friends who have quit and ask for their advice on methods and local support groups or quit-smoking programs. If it's exercise he's after and he plans to work out at home, gather advice on what to look for when buying exercise equipment, and help him shop. Or if he wants to join a health club, visit local gyms with him so that he has someone with whom to mull over his options before making a choice.

Action

This is the stage in which the person actually takes action to change his behavior.

What you can do If the plan is to reduce fat and cholesterol in the family's diet, take your partner grocery shopping. If he's not familiar with your local market, show him where the health-food aisle is. Spend some time together checking out what's there, and pick a few promising items to buy and try.

If your partner needs time to change his habit—time to attend a smoking cessation group, time to work out, time to meditate—try to arrange your own schedule to allow him that time without his feeling pressed or guilty. If it means you'll have to feed and bathe all three children by yourself two nights a week, make that commitment.

Maintenance

When the person reaches this point, he has achieved his goal and wants to continue the behavior that got him there.

What you can do Stay enthusiastic. Keep trying new low-fat recipes. Suggest a new activity you can do together to vary your exercise routines. Give him lots of compliments—about his smoke-free breath, about his appearance, about his stamina.

Lapse

Lapse is a temporary abandonment of the positive behavior followed by a quick return to it.

What you can do Don't nag. Remain supportive. Don't make your partner feel that you think this is the end of his habit change. For example, avoid negative statements like: "Well, I never thought you'd keep it up, anyway." Don't give your man the hairy eyeball when he misses a workout or has a double cheeseburger. Tell him you think it's perfectly natural to overeat during the holidays, and that it's okay to take a break from exercise periodically. Downplay the importance of the cigarettes he smoked at a friend's bachelor party if afterwards he once again becomes smoke-free.

Relapse

If a lapse goes on long enough that all the gains that were achieved disappear, the person is in relapse. To get out of relapse, he'll have to figure out what went wrong, then start over again at the contemplation stage.

What you can do Remember that even if relapse occurs, over the long haul change is still possible. Remind your partner that what he learned from this attempt will help him be successful when he's ready to try again.

Permanent Maintenance

The person in this stage has moved beyond the threat of relapse and made a permanent behavior change.

What you can do Your job is done! Just continue to be supportive, and keep that positive reinforcement coming.

PINPOINT YOUR PARTNER'S MOTIVATION STAGE

The following set of questions was designed by psychologist James O. Prochaska, Ph.D., to give people a simple way to assess their motivational stage. Identifying your partner's stage is an important first step toward helping him adopt healthier habits.

Ask your partner which of the following statements best reflects his current attitude toward the behavior(s) in question. (To avoid being repetitious, we have used only one example—adopting a low-fat diet. Just substitute the behavior your partner needs to modify.) When you've finished here, check back in "The Steps Toward Change," beginning on page 14, for a description of each stage and information on what you can do to facilitate your partner's progression to the next stage.

1. I'm not on a low-fat diet and I don't intend to adopt one in the next six months.
2. I'm not on a low-fat diet, but I intend to adopt one in the next six months.
3. I'm not on a low-fat diet, but I intend to adopt one in the next month.
4. I have been on a low-fat diet for less than the past six months.
5. I have been on a low-fat diet for more than the past six months.

Key:

If Your Partner Answered	He's at This Stage
1	Precontemplation
2	Contemplation
3	Preparation
4	Action
5	Maintenance

Encouraging the Right Kind of Motivation

Researchers talk about different types of motivation, namely positive and negative; internal and external.

Although both positive and negative motivation may work in the short term, researchers believe that to have staying power, the motivation behind a habit change has to be based on the positive consequences of that change. In other words, the perceived benefit of the change should not be simply the avoidance of negative consequences.

For example, a man who quits drinking because he's tired of not being in control of his life and wants to set a better example for his children is more likely to succeed in the long run than a man who quits drinking because his father developed cirrhosis of the liver.

This theory is supported by the fact that only 50 percent of smokers who have a heart attack stop smoking, even though cigarette smoking is known to cause heart attacks. It appears that fear—a negative emotion—isn't enough to motivate people to quit smoking, even though their lives are at stake.

One reason fear doesn't work in the long run for many people is that they forget. If a man has a heart attack or someone in his family dies of a disease that could have been prevented, his initial motivation to avoid the same fate will be strong. But as time passes, the event that triggered his decision to change will be less prominent in his mind. He would be better off if he were to quit smoking to keep up with his teammates on the basketball court (assuming he plays regularly).

As mentioned, for almost everyone, the only way motivation will last in the long term is if it comes from within. So a man who loses weight because he wants to look better in his jeans (intrinsic motivation) is more likely to lose weight and keep it off than a man who tries to lose weight because his wife wants him to look better in his jeans (extrinsic motivation).

Motivation from Within

Wanting to feel good physically and wanting to feel good about yourself and the way you look are the most productive motivators. For most people, wanting to look better just to impress the outside world won't work in the long run. Why? Because motivation that comes from outside the self is often based on guilt feelings: "I ought to do this for someone else," rather than "I want to do this for me." Extrinsic motivation usually leads to resentment, frustration, anger, and finally, quitting.

Many motivation experts suggest that before undertaking any change, a person should think about what he or she wants most from life. This kind of thinking leads to spending time on that all-important activity in behavior change: goal-setting. We'll come back to that later on.

If your partner truly understands what's essential to his well-being, he'll be able to find the motivational thoughts and feelings that will be most effective for him. For example, if a man values his family above all else, he can motivate himself to change unhealthy behavior by concentrating on how his change will improve his family life—for himself as well as for you and your children. Most likely, adopting healthier habits will improve the quality of the time he spends with his family. In addition, he'll be setting a good example for his children by teaching them to value their health and act accordingly. Likewise, if a man has work-related goals that are important to him, he can think about how changing unhealthy habits will help him accomplish those goals.

Exercising, eating right, not smoking, not drinking excessively, adhering to preventive screening guidelines—all these can help a man perform better at work, at home and at play. All your partner has to do is to see the connection between his health and what he wants to accomplish in his life. Then he can define his goals for healthy living in ways that are truly meaningful to him.

Understanding Your Man

This section is devoted to summarizing the differences between men and women in terms of how they think about health, what they value, and how they communicate. Taking the time to understand these differences will help you choose the approach that's most likely to lead to a positive response from your partner.

Of course, any described difference between the sexes is a generalization. These statements aren't true for every man and every woman. Still, researchers have found that they're true often enough to provide insights that will help the sexes understand each other a little better.

If you're like many women, you feel comfortable talking openly about health issues and are likely to seek professional help if you experience troubling symptoms. Men, on the other hand, tend to rationalize pain and discomfort, and downplay their possible causes. According to 1,500 doctors surveyed by the Men's Health Network, male patients are more likely to wait until a problem that could have been prevented or easily treated is severe or life-threatening before seeking medical help.

Some psychologists believe that this difference in attitudes toward health care comes down to the way boys and girls are raised. For example, more so than girls, boys are taught that they shouldn't cry if they get hurt. Instead, they're encouraged to get up and get on with the game. The message is that giving in to your body's signals is a sign of weakness.

While society has no problem with vulnerable women (in fact, it seems to prefer them), it scorns vulnerable men. So men do their best to be, or at least appear to be, invulnerable. One way they do that is by avoiding doctors and preventive screenings, both of which remind them of their mortality. (Men make 150 million fewer visits to the doctor a year than women do, and fully one-third of American men don't get an annual periodic health exam.)

Another way men downplay their physical vulnerability is by living a lifestyle that doesn't acknowledge that the human body needs to be taken care of. Men who pay no attention to the effect that their behavior has on their health are sending a message to the world: "I'm so tough that nothing's going to happen to me—even if I abuse my body with cigarettes, high-fat foods, and inactivity."

Women, who don't have the same need to appear invulnerable, are free to express concern about their health and that of their partners, friends, and families. You can use that freedom to help your man get healthy.

How to Talk to a Martian

When it comes to helping someone else unblock their motivation, approach is everything. How you say something and when you say it play a pivotal role in whether your statement is heard as helpful or hurtful.

Men and women have different communication styles. That means you can't completely trust your first instinct about how and when to bring up the subject of your partner's unhealthy habits. The way you communicate with other women may not be the best way to communicate with your man. As Deborah Tannen, Ph.D., puts it in her book *You Just Don't Understand—Women and Men in Conversation*, men and women "are tuned to different frequencies."

In his book, *Men are from Mars, Women are from Venus*, John Gray, Ph.D., uses a story about Martians (who represent men) and Venutians (who represent women) to explain certain differences between the sexes. According to Gray, men value power, competency, efficiency, and achievement. "Their sense of self is defined through their ability to achieve results," he writes. "Achieving goals is very important to a Martian because it's the way for him to prove his competence and thus feel good about himself. For him to feel good about himself, he must achieve these goals alone, by himself. Autonomy is a symbol of efficiency, power and competence. . . . Asking for help when you can do it yourself is a sign of weakness."

Gray goes on to explain that men tend to view unsolicited advice as criticism. Women have a hard time understanding this reaction because they view the giving of advice—solicited or not—as a show of love and support.

While self-reliance and independence are of utmost importance to men, women value community and intimacy. A woman is likely to appreciate *any* helpful advice because it makes her feel loved. A man, on the other hand, may be insulted by advice that he didn't ask for because it makes him feel inferior. The offering of unrequested advice says to a man: "I don't think you're capable of doing this on your own, so I'm offering help."

It's easy to see how this difference can create problems for women who are trying to give their men advice about living a healthier life. Here are two examples that show the difference between the way men and women perceive advice—and how that difference can cause trouble.

1. *What she says:* "I'm sorry to hear that your back is bothering you again. I just read an article that said excess weight can really strain your back. If you just cut out a few high-fat foods, like cheese, potato chips, and whole milk, I bet you could lose 15 pounds pretty easily." *What he hears:* "You're fat, and it's your fault that your back hurts." *What she meant and how she could have put it better:* "Honey, I may have found a solution to your back pain. This article says that being overweight can cause the type of pain you're experiencing. If you're interested, the article has some suggestions. I want to help you because I love you."

2. *What she says:* "I'm worried about the occasional basketball games that you play with your friends. Because you're not exercising on a regular basis, I'm concerned that you'll injure yourself. Have you thought about joining a gym so that you can work out regularly? It will probably help your game, too." *What he hears:* "You're old, out of shape, and a lousy basketball player to boot." *What she meant and how she could have put it better:* "I know how much you love to play basketball and I love that you do it. I'd like to help you find a way to exercise more often. I think that being in even better shape than you are will reduce your risk of injury and make you a more competitive player, which I know is important to you. I've got a couple of ideas to share if you'd like to hear them. I want to help you because I love you."

How do you get your message across without making your man feel criticized? Start by keeping in mind what men want. According to researchers such as Gray and Tannen, respect and acceptance are what men want most. However you frame your suggestions, be sure to do so in a manner that shows both respect and acceptance.

When you're feeling frustrated with your partner's bad habits, it might be tempting to say something like, "I can't stand your smoking. I was able to give it up when we had children, why can't you?" This statement reeks of rejection and disdain—the opposite of what men want.

Instead, wait until you're feeling less angry and try to explain exactly how your partner's smoking—or other unhealthy habit—affects you. "I worry so much when I see you smoking. I'm afraid because I don't want to live my life without you. I love you. I want you to share the joy of raising our children, and I want them to have a healthy and active father for many, many years to come. I believe that you're strong enough to beat this addiction."

Having said that many men don't like to receive unsolicited advice, it's important to point out that they do appreciate getting help when they ask for it. But here again, gender differences can cause trouble. When men confide in someone about a problem, they're looking for solutions, not sympathy. Women, on the other hand, are usually seeking empathy and understanding when they talk about a problem.

Michelle Bromley is a nutrition counselor for a diet center in South Carolina. She has noticed a definite difference between the attitudes of women and men toward losing weight. "Women need a lot of emotional support," she says. "They want to talk about how the diet is going for them and they want me to empathize with their experience."

"Men are far less emotional about dieting than women," she continues. "People on our program spend about $65 a week on food. For the men, that makes losing weight a financial issue. They're determined to get what they're paying for, so they're more focused. They don't want support. They come in, get weighed, and pick up their food for the next week."

Watch Your Language

So when talking to your partner about health habits, keep in mind that most men are primarily interested in respect, acceptance, and solutions. Although empathy might make *you* feel better by making you feel connected, it may well make your partner feel dependent—something he wants to avoid at all costs.

Phrase your suggestions so that they won't be perceived as corrections. Being careful not to hurt your man's sense of competency or threaten his independence will increase the odds that he'll accept your ideas.

Another key to effective communication is to avoid nagging, which infantilizes the person to whom you're speaking. Talking to your partner as if he were a child is likely to promote a rebellious, childlike response. Even if he wants to cooperate with you, he may feel forced into a negative reaction if you take a domineering approach.

Gray advises women to use "will" instead of "can" when asking their partner to do something. For our purposes, that might mean saying: "Honey, do you think that you *will* try to lose some weight?" instead of "Honey, do you think that you *can* lose some weight?"

What's the difference? "Will" implies a choice; "can" implies a challenge. "Will" means: Do you choose to? "Can" means: Are you able to? Most men respond better to suggestions that begin with "will" because that word sends a subtle, but important message: that *you* believe he's capable of changing if he wants to.

Six Ways to Help Your Man Get Motivated

Now that you have a better understanding of both the psychology of motivation and the psychology of men, let's look at specific motivational approaches that do and don't work. Note that each of the recommended strategies is positive—there are no criticisms or threats here. The only underlying messages are respect, acceptance, and love.

1. Share what you read about health. When you come across a relevant health article from a reliable source, share it with your partner. The trick is to avoid sounding superior. For example, don't say: "Here, *you* should read this." Instead, try saying something like this: "I read an interesting article today about dietary fiber. Apparently, it protects against heart disease and some cancers. Right now, we don't eat as much as the experts are recommending. The article lists some ways to increase fiber intake that look relatively painless. Will you read it and tell me what you think?"

2. Lead by example. Let's face it. None of us is perfect. If you're like most Americans, there are probably some habits of your own that could be changed for the healthier. Talk about what you'd like to change in your own life, share your goals, and let your partner see you work toward them. Even if your weight is perfect for your height, your diet might need some fine-tuning. Perhaps you don't eat the recommended five servings of fruits and vegetables a day, or perhaps your diet is too high in fat. If you set about to improve your diet, your partner is bound to improve his as well.

If your partner smokes or drinks too much, take a look at your own habits. If you both enjoy a glass of wine with dinner, but he keeps going with two more, you may need to give up your one glass. Many people find it's not as much fun to drink alone. Naturally, if you're a smoker and you want your partner to quit, you'll have to quit, too.

3. Make changing a team effort. Rather than putting all the emphasis on what your partner needs to do to get healthier, cast the whole thing as an adventure for the two of you. If your partner has slipped into a sedentary state, help him get the jump start he needs by organizing an active vacation or weekend getaway. Plan to run a 5K race and get in shape together. Compare feelings—both physical and emotional—along the way.

If you're already in shape, don't leave your man to get started on his own. Bear in mind, however, that if he has been inactive, inviting him to tag along on your usual five-mile run isn't a good idea. He won't be able to keep up, and that will be a discouraging blow to his ego. Instead, vary your routine to include a workout that's new to both of you. Perhaps you can both take up cycling, canoeing, weight lifting, or fast walking.

4. Rethink your social life. If your social life consists of meeting friends at restaurants, where all there is to do is drink, smoke and eat fat-laden appetizers, try some new activities. Team up with friends who are interested in adopting a healthier lifestyle, and try new things together. Check out a local theater. (In many towns, you can see a live performance for just a little more than the price of a movie ticket.) Try a concert that takes place in an auditorium or concert hall rather than a bar. Meet friends for a hike instead of a beer. Plan a family evening: take your children to a movie or an amusement park.

5. Boost his self-esteem. In his studies of dieters, David Black, associate professor of health promotion at Purdue University, has found that giving "self-esteem support" is the most effective way one person can help another lose weight. Unfortunately, people who try to help a partner change his or her habits tend to do the opposite: they act as the bad-habit police, pointing out every misstep that's made. Black found that type of help to be no help at all. Dieters did much better when their partners offered compliments and expressions of pride in their progress. You can offer positive comments right from the start. Even when little or no progress has been made, you might compliment your partner's resolve or his positive attitude.

6. Show your man that he's in control. Your role is to help your partner take control of his behavior, not to try to control it for him. For many people, taking control is central to both starting a habit change and sticking with it.

Recognizing and making choices are the chief ways to gain a sense of control. If your partner is thinking about starting an exercise program, discuss his choices with him.

Will he work out in a gym or outside? Will he work out alone or with friends? Will he try a new sport or an old favorite?

If your mate is having trouble getting started, suggest a simple and painless change rather than pushing him to tackle his biggest problem right away. His success will show him that he *can* control his behavior and encourage him to continue. For example, if your man's diet needs a major overhaul, start by suggesting a simple improvement, like eating one piece of fruit a day. Realize that he may not make even that small change right away. But the thought that you've put in his head could be the one that bumps him up a stage in the motivational process. Once he starts thinking about his eating habits, it probably won't be long before he becomes aware that they aren't healthy. That's significant progress.

Taking simple but meaningful steps toward change sets your partner up for success, rather than failure. Even small successes will make it clear to your partner that he has control over his own behavior. When your partner starts considering other, more difficult changes, you can remind him of his previous accomplishments.

Whether you choose one or all of the preceding approaches, remember the pleasure principle. People are more likely to try—and stick to—any habit change if it offers pleasure. The simple fact that changing an unhealthy habit can keep one alive longer isn't enough to motivate most people. You must find—and point out to your partner—the pleasurable aspects of any new habit you want him to adopt.

For example, let's say your partner's mind is on his work 12 or more hours a day, at home as well as in the office, and that the resulting stress is having a negative effect on

his health and your relationship. To encourage him to create time apart from work for himself and for his family,
suggest that he stop checking voice mail from home. Or
propose that he stay at work an extra half hour each night
to tie up loose ends so that he won't be tempted to do so
from home. Then point out the pleasurable side-effects of
the change: By separating his professional and personal
lives, he'll be able to focus more fully on each. Maybe he'll
actually get around to building the deck he's been planning. And, taking a complete break from work each evening will certainly make him more productive on the job.

MOTIVATION, INTERNET STYLE

Does your man enjoy checking out all that the Internet has to offer?
If so, he may find this Web site helpful: http://www.medaccess.
com. In addition to current health information, this site offers MedAccess
Motivator, a "personalized work book and on-line record keeper." The Motivator is designed to help users meet their goals in losing weight, managing
stress, exercising, eating better, and quitting smoking. It creates customized
meal and exercise plans, charts the user's daily progress, and provides support
through motivational messages. In addition to the Motivator, the MedAccess
Web site offers a bimonthly health newsletter, health quizzes, and links to
physician databases.

The Tactless Tactics

Having said what you can do to mobilize your man's motivation, let's look at some tactics that are almost certain to
backfire. We call them the tactless tactics. They have one
thing in common: They're likely to make your partner less
inclined, rather than more inclined, to be open to your
suggestions and advice. Why? Because they're all forms of

criticism and guilt promotion, and no one likes to be criticized or made to feel guilty.

- **The statistical tactic.** "250,000 people die each year for lack of physical exercise. Do you want to be one of them?" This approach makes the problem being discussed seem remote. "Yes, lack of exercise is a problem for some people in this country," your man may reason, "but not for me. I feel great."

Even if your man does feel that his sedentary lifestyle is a problem, this frightening statistic will repel him rather than attract him to your agenda. It boils down to the pleasure principle. Exercising because you enjoy the activity you've chosen, or because you enjoy the time alone, is pleasurable. But exercising because you think you might die if you don't is a burden.

- **The hands-off tactic.** "It's your body. Ruin it if you want to." This type of statement says, essentially, that you've given up on your partner and that you don't care anymore about his health and well-being. Expect him to withdraw and to feel defensive, defiant, and hurt—all of which will hinder rather than help your cause. "You're damn right it's my body," he might respond, "and it's fine the way it is. You should love me just the way I am."

- **The guilt tactic.** "Our son has asthma and I'm at risk for lung cancer because *you* smoke." Although what you're saying may well be true, your partner is likely to think you're exaggerating. In any case, he'll certainly resent being blamed for your son's illness. Guilt doesn't make people feel motivated, it just makes them feel guilty.

- **The "you're not the man you used to be" tactic.** Women using this approach usually rely on a picture to do their talking for them. The picture—one of the man in question when he weighed 30 to 40 (or more) pounds less than he does today—is taped to the refrigerator door, ostensibly to motivate the man to stay out of said appliance. What does this accomplish? Usually, it just reminds the man of how far he has to go, which makes him want to give up. It also may make him think you find him unattractive, a feeling that's more likely to dishearten than to motivate.

• **The punitive tactic.** Threats such as: "If you don't stop smoking, I'll leave you" usually have the opposite of their intended effect. When a man hears this, he feels he's under attack and usually responds by fighting back. If he agrees to give up cigarettes under these circumstances, the change is unlikely to stick. Why? He won't be changing because he decided to, but because you decided he should.

Of course, there are exceptions. A threat from a female partner can bring about lasting change if the woman means what she says 100 percent. In other words, when a woman is totally prepared to act on her threat, it may be perceived as a statement of fact rather than a threat.

Telling your partner what the consequences of his continued disregard for his health will be can make the problem more real to him. For example, a man who isn't motivated by a concern—yours or his—that he might eventually get sick because of his behavior, may be motivated to change by a more immediate threat to his happiness.

After Bob Meade recovered from his first heart attack, he continued to smoke cigarettes when he was away from home. He did so even though his doctor had told him that his habit of smoking two packs a day probably caused his heart attack.

More than once, Ava Meade smelled cigarette smoke on Bob when he got home. "I told him: 'If I ever smell smoke on you again, the kids and I are leaving,'" recalls Ava. She explains that she wasn't willing to put herself or her children through the agony of watching him contribute to his own demise. "The children were scared to death by the first heart attack," she says. "I didn't want them to have to go through that—or worse—again.

"They tell you in the rehabilitation program [for heart attack survivors] not to threaten," Ava continues. "But I wasn't threatening. I meant it. I was prepared to leave if he continued smoking." Bob hasn't smoked since.

Getting Started

Your partner may not think he has a problem behavior, regardless of how obvious it seems to you. If that's the case, your call for change is likely to fall on deaf ears. Marc Tallent, Ph.D., a clinical psychologist in New York City, recommends approaching the subject of a man's unhealthy habits by first finding out about his perception of the problem.

In other words, don't start your discussion with a statement like: "You need to go on a diet and get on a treadmill." That's jumping to a solution before you've agreed there's a problem. Instead, tell your partner that you're concerned about his unhealthy habit. You'll quickly know whether he understands your concern or thinks it's unfounded. (If your partner has several unhealthy habits, stick to the one that's likely having the most detrimental effect on his health for now. Trying to tackle a list of unhealthy habits all at once will probably discourage you both. And, as we have pointed out, making one change can help the person to make another, and then another.)

Often, getting a man to admit that his habits are problematic is a matter of education. As discussed earlier, men don't talk or read about health as much as women do. Your partner may not realize how important exercise is. He may not understand how his diet affects his heart.

Dr. Tallent suggests asking your partner: "Do you want to know why I'm concerned about your diet (smoking, lack of exercise, drinking)? I'd like to talk about it when you're ready." Getting your partner's permission to talk about the issue shows respect and acceptance. The opposite approach, rattling off facts and dire predictions about his life span whether he wants to hear it or not, will make him feel like a child being scolded.

Don't Overwhelm Him

Once you get permission to share your concerns, don't overwhelm your partner with a lot of information. Plant the idea with a few simple statements, then feed him more facts periodically, allowing him time to think about each new piece of information. Follow up by asking whether he's had a chance to think about what you discussed.

Let's say that your partner subsists mainly on fast food and ice cream, despite the fact that his father died of a heart attack at the age of 55. Start your campaign by explaining that your partner's family history puts him at risk for heart disease, then mention that diet and exercise can help reduce his risk. Your message should be: "I love you and want you around." On another day, you might share an article from the newspaper that explains the role of cholesterol in heart disease—and so on.

Dr. Tallent emphasizes that sometimes a seemingly

straightforward problem, like overeating, isn't as simple as it appears. Unhealthy behavior can be the manifestation of an emotional problem that needs to be resolved before the behavior can be changed.

"Self-destructive behaviors can be a way of acting out against a spouse," says Dr. Tallent. "They can be a way of handling anger inappropriately." Some such problems can be addressed by the couple; others may benefit from professional help to untangle the emotions, grudges, and misunderstandings that have accumulated.

"I've seen people who've had angioplasty and bypass surgery who continue to eat foods that are bad for their hearts," says Dr. Tallent. "In cases like that, it may be helpful for the man or the couple to talk to someone outside the relationship to find out what's behind that behavior."

The bottom line is that you should realize that unhealthy behavior can be a sensitive issue. One accusing word can trigger a defensive reaction that will drastically reduce your chances of helping your man get healthier. "If you talk about eating habits, your partner may hear your comments as extreme criticism or as an expression of love, depending on how you phrase it," says Dr. Tallent. "Broaching the topic in the wrong way is worse than not broaching it at all. It can set you back even farther by making your partner resist your point of view."

Once your partner has agreed that he'd like to change, he'll need to set specific goals. Research shows that having a well-defined, realistic goal significantly increases the likelihood that a person will accomplish the changes for which he's aiming. Research also shows that people who share their goals with supportive friends and family are more likely to stick to their plans, so encourage your man to open up.

HOW HEALTHY ARE YOUR HABITS?

Take this quiz with your partner. Use it as a springboard for a discussion of how you could both improve your habits and lifestyle choices.

Circle the letter to the left of the answer that best describes you. Use the following scoring key: A = 1; B = 2; C = 3; D = 4; E = 5.

1. I eat red meat the following number of times per week:
   A. 7 or more
   B. 5 or 6
   C. 4
   D. 2 or 3
   E. 0 or 1
   Score:_____

2. The following represents the approximate number of pounds I weigh over my ideal body weight:
   A. 30 lbs.
   B. 20 lbs.
   C. 10 lbs.
   D. 5 lbs.
   E. I am at my ideal weight.
   Score:_____

Here's a quick way to determine ideal weight. For a man, start with 110 pounds and add 6 pounds for every inch of height above 5 feet. For a woman, start with 100 pounds and add 5 pounds for every inch of height above 5 feet.

3. I exercise:
   A. Never
   B. Occasionally
   C. Once a month
   D. Two or three times a month
   E. Five times a week
   Score:_____

4. I usually have the following number of drinks each day:
    A. More than 8
    B. 6–8
    C. 4–5
    D. 3
    E. 0–2
    Score:_____

5. My exercise routine lasts:
    A. I never exercise
    B. 10 minutes
    C. 15 minutes
    D. 30 minutes
    E. 45 minutes to an hour
    Score:_____

6. When I wake up in the morning, I am:
    A. Unable to get out of bed
    B. Extremely fatigued and groggy
    C. Tired but able to function well
    D. A bit sleepy but ready to go
    E. Well rested, alert and looking forward to the day
    Score:_____

7. In times of stress, I generally:
    A. Blame others and get angry
    B. Feel debilitated and immobilized
    C. Avoid the situation and walk away
    D. Try to stay calm and cope
    E. Manage the challenge
    Score:_____

8. My overall attitude toward life is:
   A. Bleak and extremely dissatisfied
   B. Generally pessimistic
   C. Indifferent
   D. Content
   E. Enthusiastic
   Score:_____

9. In my daily life I generally get:
   A. Negative input from others
   B. Indifference from others
   C. Limited support from others
   D. Professional and personal support
   E. A broad base of constructive support
   Score:_____

10. I go to the doctor:
    A. Never, or only in an emergency
    B. When I feel very sick
    C. When someone forces me to go
    D. When I don't feel well
    E. Routinely
    Score:_____

Total Score:_____

What Your Score Means

41–50 High score wins! You have excellent health-management skills.

31–40 Keep up the good work. Is there any single category where you could work a little harder?

21–30 You need to pay more attention to your health management. Where do you need to make improvements? Check your scores and make a list of areas that would benefit from closer attention. Then take it step by step.

11–20 Improving your health-management skills will require some behavior modification. Build on your strengths. For example, if you occasionally exercise but are overweight, work toward exercising on a regular basis. Ask your doctor or a nutritionist for advice on how to adopt a healthier diet.

1–10 A wake-up call. It's time to start paying attention to your health and manage it as you would your bank account. Your health professionals can help you get started. Line up some support for change.

Adapted with permission from the New York City Health and Hospitals Corporation Healthy Habits and Choices © 1996

Help Your Man Set Reachable Goals

People have a number of ingenious ways of sabotaging their efforts at reform. As you listen to your partner's goals, watch out for these common pitfalls:

• **Setting unrealistic goals.** "I've been thinking about that program we watched together on heart disease. I've decided I really need to lose fifty pounds. I'm going to do it in six months, before your sister's wedding." While these may be the words you've been longing to hear, they should sound little alarm bells in your head. Fifty pounds is a lot of weight—even for someone who weighs 300 pounds. And six months is hardly enough time to lose that kind of weight without a crash diet. Even if that goal is reached with a crash diet, the likelihood of maintaining the weight loss is slim. Remember, your goal is to encourage permanent changes in diet, exercise and other habits that, together, will make your partner healthier—not to have him looking good at your sister's wedding, only to fall back to the unhealthy habits soon after.

Deep down inside, your partner may wish he looked like Arnold Schwarzenegger, but chances are that's not a realistic goal. There's a strong genetic component in body shape and size and in determining whether you can, for example, significantly increase the bulk of your muscles. The goals your partner sets for himself should suit *him*.

If your partner needs to lose weight, discourage him from thinking in terms of a movie-star physique. Getting *thin* isn't the only way to improve health—getting thin*ner* works wonders for many. Losing 10 percent of body weight—and keeping it off—is a realistic goal that will enhance health for most people.

• **Setting too many goals.** "You're right honey, I've been neglecting my health for too long," your partner says one day. You hold your breath. Is he really finally ready to change? "I'm going to join the gym, quit smoking and lose 20 pounds. Throw out all the potato chips and pizza." If you're smart, you'll slow him down. Making all of those changes at once is certain to tax his will power and lead to failure on all counts. Suggest that he try one change at a time.

• **Setting goals that aren't specific.** To act on a goal, you need to know exactly what would constitute reaching the goal. For example, if your partner sets a goal to "ride my bike more often," how will he measure his compliance? How much, exactly, is "more often"? He would have a better chance for success if his goal were to "ride my bike five miles every day."

- **Failing to recognize—and reward—small successes.** Encourage your partner to pat himself on the back for every benchmark. One week without cigarettes? Ask him out to the movies—his choice. A month smoke-free? Suggest that he buy himself that new drill he's been eyeing.

- **Using negative motivators.** Research shows that people who are motivated by negative thoughts are less likely to achieve long-lasting success than those who are motivated by positive thoughts. Although negative thoughts can work well initially, helping your partner convert his negative motivations to positive ones will improve his chances of success.

Let's say, for example, that your partner stopped smoking because his grandfather was diagnosed with lung cancer. He has been smoke-free for a month. It's time encourage your partner to begin focusing on the positive reasons for quitting. Point out that not smoking gives your partner more energy, improves his health, helps him save a little extra money, gives him fresher breath, and helps him keep up with the guys on his flag-football team.

Some scientists spend their careers studying the psychology of how people change and improve themselves. When you start looking at what one person can do to help motivate another, the issues grow even more complex. So you may want to reread this chapter—or parts of it—periodically. An understanding of motivation and how it works will help you in your own life, too.

TEN WAYS TO BOOST YOUR MATE'S MOTIVATION

1. Tell him you love him.
2. Share relevant health information.
3. Set a good example.
4. Point out small successes.
5. Ignore small failures.
6. Speak with respect.
7. Encourage him to share his goals.
8. Help him find positive reasons for change.
9. Help him avoid temptation.
10. Tell him you love him.

2

SHARE THE WORD ON SCREENING

> *After death, the doctor.*
>
> *George Herbert*

Every year, men make 150 million fewer visits to doctors than women. This disparity occurs at every age, *not* just in the childbearing years (women have about 12 prenatal visits per pregnancy). Why is it that so many men would prefer, as George Herbert so succinctly said, to put off seeing a doctor until they need a death certificate?

"Men really detest going to the doctor," says Michael Lafavore, editor-in-chief of *Men's Health,* a magazine with 1.5 million (mostly male) readers. "It's really amazing what lengths they'll go to to avoid physicians. Even if a man is hurting bad, he may not seek medical care."

Lafavore cites the death of Jim Henson as an example. Henson suffered with severe invasive strep A, the infamous flesh-eating bacteria, for several days. When he finally went to the hospital, he took a cab rather than calling an ambulance. By the time he sought care, it was too late.

An American Medical Association study concluded that men don't go to the doctor for four main reasons: fear, denial, embarrassment, and threatened masculinity. Let's look at each of those factors in turn.

Fear and **denial** go hand in hand. Men who avoid doctors do so at least in part because they fear bad news. "If I don't see a doctor for a routine physical," the thinking goes, "he can't find anything wrong with me." Denial further encourages the fearful to avoid doctors. "I feel fine, therefore I am fine—and if I'm not fine, I don't want to know about it."

As for plain old **embarrassment,** in one survey one out of 10 men said they'd rather undergo root-canal surgery than have a digital rectal exam to check for prostate cancer. In another study, 20 percent of men surveyed said that embarrassment might stop them from talking about prostate or colorectal problems, which in turn, could stop them from receiving early treatment, which is most effective.

Finally, there's the **masculinity** issue. "A doctor is someone in a position of authority," says Lafavore. "You have to humble yourself. The doctor may keep you waiting, and may well perform some disagreeable examinations. All in all, the whole experience is detrimental to a man's feelings of masculinity."

Real Men Don't Need Doctors

In addition, some men view having a health problem as a sign of weakness. "Men are very competitive with each other," says Lafavore. "We don't want anybody to have an advantage over us. If at all possible, we don't take sick days, and we avoid having medical appointments that cause us to arrive to work late or leave early."

The bottom line, says Lafavore: "Women have to be aware that some men will find every excuse *not* to go to the doctor."

Ava Meade, whose husband, Bob, had his first heart attack when he was just shy of 34, agrees: "Men can be very stubborn about going to the doctor," she says. "I go for my Pap smear every year. I don't like going, but I do. A lot of men have a real aversion to being reminded of their mortality."

Bob's first heart attack occurred the evening after a racquetball game. During the game, he didn't feel well and stopped playing, but by the time he got home he felt better and didn't want to see a doctor. "I took one look at him and said: 'Something's wrong,'" remembers Ava. "We took him kicking and screaming to the hospital. He was admitted for observation and hooked up to a heart monitor. The nurses woke him up in the middle of the night and said: 'You're having a heart attack.'"

It was a silent (symptomless) heart attack, the kind that accounts for somewhere between 25 and 40 percent of all myocardial infarctions (the medical term for "heart attack"). An angioplasty was performed. (Angioplasty is a procedure in which a catheter—a thin, flexible tube—with a balloon tip is inserted in an artery in the groin or arm. The catheter is then threaded into the coronary arteries and, when it reaches an area congested with plaque, the balloon tip is inflated to open up the blockage.) Within a year, Bob asked to be taken off the medication that was helping to keep his arteries dilated (open). "He was in a lot of denial," says Ava. "He hated taking medication. It reminded him that there was something wrong with him."

Then one Spring Saturday in 1994, Bob again didn't feel well. He called his doctor's office, and the physician on-call told him to start taking his medication again. Bob decided to wait until Monday, when he could speak to his personal physician. He had his second heart attack on Sunday night.

"He woke me up and said he felt like he was choking and that his throat hurt," recalls Ava. "I called the paramedics and followed them to the hospital, where a cardiogram confirmed that Bob had had another heart attack."

Having two heart attacks convinced Bob that he might need doctors more than he had previously liked to admit. "I used to beg him to go for a physical," says Ava. "Now, he keeps all of his appointments and he goes in with his mouth closed. He's more humble."

A PREVENTIVE SCREENING SCHEDULE FOR MEN

Okay, so you've convinced your man of the importance of preventive health care. But exactly what examinations, tests, and shots does he need, and when? The following schedule was put together using recommendations from several sources, including the American Cancer Society, the American Diabetes Association, and the Men's Health Clinic in Dallas, Texas. Your doctor may use a slightly different schedule. If so, it's best to go with hers or his. But the commonly used schedules today are generally in the same ballpark.

Age	Recommended Preventive Care (frequency)
20–39	Blood pressure (every year); Health-risk appraisal, including blood and urine tests (every 3 years); Tuberculosis antibody test (every 5 years); Electrocardiogram, if at high risk for heart attack (every 3 to 5 years); Tetanus booster (every 10 years).
40–49	Blood pressure (every year); Rectal exam (every year); prostate-specific antigen (PSA) blood test, if at high risk for prostate cancer (every year); Health-risk appraisal, including blood and urine tests (every 2 years); blood-sugar test (first at age 45—earlier if at high risk—and every 3 years thereafter); Electrocardiogram, if at high risk for heart attack (every 3 to 5 years); Tetanus booster (every 10 years).

50 plus   Blood pressure (every year); Health-risk appraisal, including blood and urine tests (every year); Rectal exam (every year); PSA blood test (every year); Hemoccult test (every year); Blood-sugar test (every 3 years); Sigmoidoscopy (every 3 to 5 years); Electrocardiogram (every 3 to 5 years); Tetanus booster (every 10 years).

How You Can Help

Education is an important first step in your campaign to get your man the preventive care he needs. Read up together on what each test or exam entails and how it can help protect a man's health. This will help your partner see that following preventive care guidelines is well worth the effort of getting to a doctor's office once a year (at most)—and even well worth enduring the dreaded digital rectal exam.

The following is a rundown of the tests and exams your man can expect his physician to recommend. We start with prostate-cancer screening—and talk a lot about it—because one of its components is quite controversial, and because prostate cancer may well be the disease men fear most.

Prostate-Cancer Screening

Two tests are commonly recommended to help ensure that prostate cancer, if present, is detected early enough to be treated successfully. The digital rectal exam (DRE) is a physical exam performed by a physician. He or she inserts a lubricated, gloved finger into the rectum and gently feels for bumps or abnormal areas in and on the rectal lining. The doctor also will feel the prostate through the wall of the rectum to check for abnormalities. The exam may cause mild discomfort, but shouldn't cause pain.

The second test used to screen for prostate cancer is the PSA blood test. PSA stands for prostate-specific antigen, which is a protein made only by the prostate. When there's cancer in the prostate, it secretes more PSA than usual. Elevated PSA levels show up in the bloodstream. However, prostate cancer comes in a variety of forms, from mild (a mild cancer is one that doesn't spread) to severe. Further, prostate cancer treatment can carry with it complications ranging from incontinence to impotence. Thus there's a great deal of controversy over how frequently men should have PSA tests for screening purposes, and whether all men need to be screened on a regular basis.

The American Cancer Society advocates annual testing for all men older than 50 who are expected to live another decade. African-American males should begin screening at age 40 because their risk of prostate cancer is 30 percent higher than the risk for white males. White males who have a family history of prostate cancer also should begin testing at age 40 because of their increased risk.

On the other hand, the American College of Physicians (ACP), a professional society representing 85,000 internists, recommends *against* annual screening for *all* men, saying that there's no evidence that all patients benefit. The organization suggests that men discuss with their physicians whether it's necessary in their particular case to have a PSA test every year.

A study done at Johns Hopkins University supports the ACP position. Researchers who studied blood samples from 40 men with prostate cancer and 272 men with no evidence of prostate cancer concluded that annual PSA testing of all men is unlikely to save lives. They suggest, instead, that men whose PSA levels are less than 2 nanograms per milliliter at the first test wait two years before having another test. The reason? Men with such low levels aren't likely to develop incurable prostate cancer before being tested again in two years. The potential cost savings of this recommendation are huge—one researcher estimates savings to be $450 million a year—because 70 percent of men aged 50 to 70 have PSA levels of less than 2.

Another strike against the PSA test is that it has a significant false-positive rate, meaning that the test sometimes indicates the presence of cancer where in reality none exists. Conditions other than cancer, such as benign prostatic hypertrophy (BPH—an enlargement of the prostate that's a common outcome of aging) or prostatitis (an infection of the prostate), also can cause the gland to secrete increased amounts of the PSA protein.

According to the Centers for Disease Control and Prevention, about 50 percent of men with benign prostatic hypertrophy have elevated PSA levels and thus may receive additional diagnostic tests for cancer, such as a biopsy (a surgical procedure in which a small bit of the prostate is removed for studying) and transrectal ultrasound. Many of the men who receive these additional tests aren't ultimately diagnosed with prostate cancer, so they've been put through an anxiety-producing, time-consuming, and costly set of tests unnecessarily.

In addition to producing false positives, the PSA test sometimes produces false negatives. That is, the test fails to detect some prostate cancer. In fact, about 20 percent of patients with biopsy-proven prostate cancer have PSA levels that fall within the normal range.

Nevertheless, the fact remains that the PSA test *can* find prostate cancer long before a physician could feel an abnormality on the prostate gland through DRE. The value of early detection through screening is supported by studies that have found locally advanced and metastatic disease (that which has spread to other organs and areas of the body) to be markedly more common among men who did not have regular screening than among men who did. In 1996, the death rate for prostate cancer dropped for the first time in more than 60 years, just eight years after the PSA test became widely used.

 SEVEN WARNING SIGNS OF CANCER
1. Change in bowel or bladder habits
2. A sore that doesn't heal
3. Unusual bleeding or discharge
4. Thickening or lumps in breast or elsewhere
   (men can get breast cancer, too, although it's rare)
5. Indigestion or difficulty in swallowing
6. Obvious change in wart or mole
7. Nagging cough or hoarseness

Source: The National Foundation for Cancer Research

Overcoming Resistance to Prostate-Cancer Screening

If your man resists the idea of an annual DRE and an annual (or biannual) PSA test, remind him that approximately 40,000 men die of prostate cancer each year in the U.S. If he's younger than 60, remind him, too, that prostate cancer isn't confined to older men. Of men age 40 to 59, one in 57 develops prostate cancer.

As you set about convincing your man that he should be diligent about prostate-cancer screening, know in advance that you might be in for a fight. According to a survey published in the *Archives of Family Medicine,* seven out of 10 husbands said they preferred *not* to undergo annual prostate cancer screening. (On the other hand, nine out of 10 wives were in favor of annual screening.) The researchers concluded that, when faced with a choice between living longer but experiencing prostate-cancer treatment complications such as impotence and incontinence, men would prefer a shorter life with no such complications. Wives, on the other hand, would prefer to have their husbands live longer, even if those complications were to occur.

If your partner sides with the majority of men on this issue, tell him about a survey of 274 Minneapolis men who had had either radical prostatectomy or radiation therapy for prostate cancer. First, the bad news: complications of the treatments were common, and *didn't* disappear with time. They included impotence (70 percent of those who had surgery and 50 percent of those who had radiation), incontinence (52 percent of the group that had surgery and 15 percent of the group that had radiation), and bowel dysfunction (8 percent of those who had surgery and 21 percent of those who had radiation). Nevertheless—and here's the important point—the average rating given by men who had surgery to the overall quality of their lives was 93.8 on a scale of 0 to 112. Those men who had radiation assigned their lives an average quality rating of 87.7. The bottom line is that despite having significant symptoms, the men reported a fairly good quality of life.

In addition, you can point out that new treatments are being developed for prostate cancer that will reduce the risk of complications such as impotence and incontinence. For example, as this book is being written, surgeons are evaluating a simple procedure that can prevent urinary incontinence in men who undergo surgical removal of the prostate. When the prostate is removed, the bladder can fall into the cavity that's created, causing incontinence. In this new procedure, tissue is used to tie the bladder into its correct place, which seems to reduce the risk of incontinence.

Also on the horizon is a way to avoid surgical damage to the microscopic nerves that surround the prostate and control sexual function. That damage causes impotence in more than half the men who have radical prostatectomy (complete surgical removal of the prostate). The Food and Drug Administration (FDA) has approved a new surgical device called "CaverMap" that uses a live electrical probe to detect critical prostatic nerves and warn surgeons when they are about to cut one. This new development may improve the success of nerve-sparing prostate surgery using older techniques, which researchers at the Massachusetts General Hospital in Boston found didn't significantly reduce postsurgical risk of impotence and actually *increased* postsurgical risk of urinary incontinence.

Blood-Pressure Screening

Blood pressure is expressed as two numbers: systolic pressure and diastolic pressure. The first is the pressure measured in the arteries when the heart contracts. The second is the lower pressure measured when the heart relaxes between beats. Blood pressure is measured in millimeters of mercury (mm Hg). Generally, hypertension is defined as systolic pressure greater than 140 mm Hg or diastolic pressure greater than 90 mm Hg (140/90 mm Hg).

To measure blood pressure, a doctor or other health professional wraps a blood-pressure cuff (a flat rubber "bladder" covered in heavy cloth) around the patient's upper arm. The bladder is pumped full of air so that blood flow in the arm is temporarily stopped. The health-care provider then listens with a stethoscope placed over an artery on the side of the cuff that's away from the heart for the return of blood flow as the cuff is gradually deflated. There's a gauge attached to a rubber tube leading to the bladder. As the blood flow returns, the pressure at which the heartbeat can first be heard is the systolic pressure. The pressure at which the sound disappears is the diastolic pressure.

In general, blood pressures above 130/85 mm Hg are considered to be at least slightly elevated and require additional investigation to determine whether intervention of one sort or another is needed. Lifestyle changes will probably be recommended to help reduce blood pressure. Medications may also be prescribed, especially if blood pressure is 160/100 mm Hg or above.

Although high blood pressure often causes no symptoms, it shouldn't be mistaken for a harmless condition—far from it. Untreated hypertension can damage the arteries and secondarily the brain, heart, and kidneys. Thus, high blood pressure is a major risk factor for stroke, heart attack, and kidney problems. Because of the potentially serious consequences of untreated hypertension, the American Heart Association recommends that blood pressure be measured in all adults at least every 2.5 years and preferably every year.

QUESTIONS DOCTORS ARE LIKELY TO ASK

This sample patient questionnaire will give your mate an idea of what he may be asked—either on paper or in person by the physician—at a doctor's visit. Suggest that your man take a look at this sample before his appointment. That way, he'll have a chance to find out the answers to health history questions he may be unsure about.

Source: Courtesy John Biasetti, M.D.

PATIENT'S NAME _____   BIRTH DATE _____   SEX _____   S.M.W.D.

ADDRESS _____   TEL. NO. _____

INSURANCE _____   REFERRED BY _____   OCCUPATION _____

INSTRUCTIONS: PUT ☑ IN THOSE BOXES APPLICABLE TO YOU AND IN THE "YES" OR "NO" SPACE. IF LINES ARE PROVIDED WRITE IN YOUR ANSWER.

FAMILY HISTORY

	FATHER	MOTHER	BROTHER				SISTER				SPOUSE	CHILDREN					
			1	2	3	4	1	2	3	4		1	2	3	4	5	6
AGE (IF LIVING)																	
HEALTH (G) GOOD (B) BAD																	
CANCER																	
TUBERCULOSIS																	
DIABETES																	
HEART TROUBLE																	
HIGH BLOOD PRESSURE																	
STROKE																	
EPILEPSY																	
NERVOUS BREAKDOWN																	
ASTHMA, HIVES, HAY FEVER																	
BLOOD DISEASE																	
AGE (AT DEATH)																	
CAUSE OF DEATH																	

PERSONAL HISTORY

HAVE YOU EVER HAD	NO	YES	HAVE YOU EVER HAD	NO	YES	HAVE YOU EVER HAD	NO	YES
☐ SCARLET FEVER ☐ SCARLATINA			☐ GONORRHEA ☐ SYPHILIS			ANY ☐ BROKEN ☐ CRACKED BONES		
DIPHTHERIA			ANEMIA			RECURRENT DISLOCATIONS		
SMALLPOX			JAUNDICE			☐ CONCUSSION ☐ HEAD INJURY		
PNEUMONIA			EPILEPSY			EVER BEEN KNOCKED UNCONSCIOUS		
PLEURISY			MIGRAINE HEADACHES			☐ FOOD ☐ CHEMICAL ☐ DRUG POISONING		

UNDULANT FEVER			TUBERCULOSIS		EXPLAIN
☐ RHEUMATIC FEVER ☐ HEART DISEASE			DIABETES		
ST. VITUS DANCE			CANCER		
☐ ARTHRITIS ☐ RHEUMATISM			☐ HIGH ☐ LOW BLOOD PRESSURE		ANY OTHER DISEASE
ANY ☐ BONE ☐ JOINT DISEASE			NERVOUS BREAKDOWN		EXPLAIN
☐ NEURITIS ☐ NEURALGIA			☐ HAY FEVER ☐ ASTHMA		
☐ BURSITIS ☐ SCIATICA ☐ LUMBAGO			☐ HIVES ☐ ECZEMA		
☐ POLIO ☐ MENINGITIS			FREQUENT ☐ COLDS ☐ SORE THROAT		WEIGHT: NOW ___ ONE YR. AGO ___
BRIGHT'S DISEASE			FREQUENT ☐ INFECTIONS ☐ BOILS		MAXIMUM ___ WHEN ___

ALLERGIES

ARE YOU ALLERGIC TO	NO	YES	ARE YOU ALLERGIC TO	NO	YES	ARE YOU ALLERGIC TO	NO	YES
☐ PENCILLIN ☐ SULFA DRUGS			ANY OTHER DRUGS			ANY FOODS		
☐ ASPIRIN ☐ CODEINE ☐ MORPHINE			EXPLAIN			EXPLAIN		
☐ MYCINS ☐ OTHER ANTIBIOTICS								
☐ TETANUS ☐ ANTITOXIN ☐ SERUMS			ADHESIVE TAPE			☐ NAIL POLISH ☐ OTHER COSMETICS		

SURGERY

HAVE YOU HAD REMOVED	NO	YES	HAVE YOU HAD REMOVED	NO	YES	HAVE YOU	NO	YES
TONSILS			☐ OVARY ☐ OVARIES			HAD HERNIA REPAIRED		
APPENDIX			HEMORRHOIDS			HAD ANY OTHER OPERATIONS		
GALL BLADDER			EVER HAVE A TRANSFUSION			BEEN HOSPITALIZED FOR ANY ILLNESS		
UTERUS			☐ BLOOD ☐ PLASMA			EXPLAIN		

X-RAYS

EVER HAVE X-RAYS OF	NO	YES	DATE	DISEASE PRESENT
CHEST				
☐ STOMACH ☐ COLON				
GALL BLADDER				
EXTREMITIES				
BACK				
OTHER				

HISTACOUNT CORPORATION, MELVILLE, N. Y. 11747

SYSTEMS

DO YOU NOW HAVE OR HAVE YOU EVER HAD	NO	YES	DO YOU NOW HAVE OR HAVE YOU EVER HAD	NO	YES
ANY □ EYE DISEASE □ EYE INJURY □ IMPAIRED SIGHT			KIDNEY □ DISEASE □ STONES		
ANY □ EAR DISEASE □ EAR INJURY □ IMPAIRED HEARING			BLADDER DISEASE		
ANY TROUBLE WITH □ NOSE □ SINUSES □ MOUTH □ THROAT			BLOOD IN URINE		
FAINTING SPELLS			□ ALBUMIN □ SUGAR □ PUS □ ETC. IN URINE		
CONVULSIONS			DIFFICULTY IN URINATION		
PARALYSIS			NARROWED URINARY STREAM		
DIZZINESS			ABNORMAL THIRST		
HEADACHES: □ FREQUENT □ SEVERE			PROSTATE TROUBLE		
ENLARGED GLANDS			□ STOMACH TROUBLE □ ULCER		
THYROID: □ OVERACTIVE □ UNDERACTIVE □ ENLARGED			INDIGESTION		
ENLARGED GOITER			□ GAS □ BELCHING		
SKIN DISEASE			APPENDICITIS		
COUGH: □ FREQUENT □ CHRONIC			□ LIVER DISEASE □ GALL BLADDER DISEASE		
□ CHEST PAIN □ ANGINA PECTORIS			□ COLITIS □ OTHER BOWEL DISEASE		
SPITTING UP BLOOD			□ HEMORRHOIDS □ RECTAL BLEEDING		
NIGHT SWEATS			BLACK TARRY STOOLS		
SHORTNESS OF BREATH □ EXERTION □ AT NIGHT			□ CONSTIPATION □ DIARRHEA		
□ PALPITATION □ FLUTTERING HEART			□ PARASITES □ WORMS		
SWELLING OF □ HANDS □ FEET □ ANKLES			□ ANY CHANGE IN APPETITE □ EATING HABITS		
VARICOSE VEINS			□ ANY CHANGE IN BOWEL ACTION □ STOOLS		
EXTREME □ TIREDNESS □ WEAKNESS			EXPLAIN		

IMMUNIZATION - EKG

HAVE YOU HAD	NO	YES	HAVE YOU HAD	NO	YES
SMALLPOX VACCINATION (WITHIN LAST 7 YEARS)			POLIO SHOTS (WITHIN LAST 2 YEARS)		
TETANUS SHOT (NOT ANTITOXIN)			AN ELECTROCARDIOGRAM WHEN		

HABITS

DO YOU.	NO	YES	DO YOU USE	NEVER	OCC.	FREQ.	DAILY
EXERCISE ADEQUATELY			LAXATIVES				
HOW?			VITAMINS				
AWAKEN RESTED			SEDATIVES				
SLEEP WELL			TRANQUILIZERS				
AVERAGE 8 HOURS SLEEP (PER NIGHT)			SLEEPING PILLS, ETC.				
HAVE REGULAR BOWEL MOVEMENTS			ASPIRINS, ETC.				
SEX - ENTIRELY SATISFACTORY			CORTISONE				
LIKE YOUR WORK (HOURS PER DAY) □ INDOORS □ OUTDOORS			ALCOHOLIC BEVERAGES				
WATCH TELEVISION (HOURS PER DAY)			COFFEE (CUPS PER DAY)				
READ (HOURS PER DAY)			TOBACCO: □ CIGARETTES (PKS PER DAY)				
HAVE A VACATION (WEEKS PER YEAR)			□ CIGARS □ PIPE □ CHEWING TOBACCO				
HAVE YOU EVER BEEN TREATED FOR ALCOHOLISM			□ SNUFF				
HAVE YOU EVER BEEN TREATED FOR DRUG ABUSE			APPETITE DEPRESSANTS				
RECREATION: DO YOU PARTICIPATE IN SPORTS OR HAVE HOBBIES WHICH GIVE YOU RELAXATION AT LEAST 3 HOURS A WEEK.			THYROID MEDICATION: □ NO □ YES, IN PAST □ NONE NOW NOW ON GR. DAILY				
			HAVE YOU EVER TAKEN . . .				
			□ INSULIN □ TABLETS FOR DIABETES □ HORMONE SHOTS □ TABLETS □ NO				

WOMEN ONLY

MENSTRUAL HISTORY	NO	YES		NO	YES
AGE AT ONSET			ARE YOU REGULAR: □ HEAVY □ MEDIUM □ LIGHT		
USUAL DURATION OF PERIOD DAYS			DO YOU HAVE □ TENSION □ DEPRESSION BEFORE PERIOD		
CYCLE (START TO START) DAYS			DO YOU HAVE □ CRAMPS □ PAIN WITH PERIODS		
DATE OF LAST PERIOD			DO YOU HAVE HOT FLASHES		
PREGNANCIES . . .	NO	YES		NO	YES
CHILDREN BORN ALIVE (HOW MANY)			STILL BORN (HOW MANY)		
CESAREAN SECTIONS (HOW MANY)			MISCARRIAGES (HOW MANY)		
PREMATURES (HOW MANY)			ANY COMPLICATIONS		

EMOTIONS

ARE YOU OFTEN	NO	YES	ARE YOU OFTEN	NO	YES
DEPRESSED			JUMPY		
ANXIOUS			JITTERY		
IRRITABLE			IS CONCENTRATION DIFFICULT?		

Cholesterol Screening

Your man's cholesterol profile can reveal a lot about his health. People with high blood levels of what's called low-density lipoprotein (LDL) cholesterol and/or high levels of another substance called triglyceride are at increased risk for heart attack and stroke. A low level of high-density lipoprotein (HDL) cholesterol—the "good" kind that carries harmful LDL cholesterol out of the body—also indicates that a person is at increased risk for heart attack and stroke. The good news is that an unhealthy cholesterol profile can be treated with lifestyle changes and/or medication. The catch is that one has to be screened to find out that one has a problem.

The National Cholesterol Education Program (run by the National Heart, Blood and Lung Institute and the American Heart Association) calls for screening total-cholesterol and HDL-cholesterol levels in all adults aged 20 and over at least every five years. Proponents of this approach say that widespread screening and subsequent intervention have contributed to the drop in cholesterol levels and heart disease in this country over the past 30 years.

However, guidelines issued by the American College of Physicians call for a more conservative approach to cholesterol screening. The ACP says that only men aged 35 to 65 and women aged 45 to 65 should be screened.

Why the fuss over a simple blood test that's recommended (by both parties) just every five years for healthy adults? According to Dr. Alan M. Garber, author of the ACP guidelines: "A chain of events is set into motion when a person is found to have high cholesterol and it too often leads to treatment through medication. These drugs haven't been tested for efficacy in young people and the long-term safety of the most popular drugs is unknown."

Still, it doesn't make a lot of sense for your man to avoid finding out his cholesterol level just because there's a risk that he might be treated unnecessarily with medication. In many cases, lifestyle changes such as losing excess weight, exercising regularly, and eating a low-fat diet can do the trick. Your man can seek a second opinion if medication is prescribed, or he can opt to try lifestyle changes alone for a certain period to see if he can improve his cholesterol profile without medication (providing, of course, that his doctor says this would be safe).

What is a healthy cholesterol profile? There are three numbers that are key players in the cholesterol story that blood has to tell. As mentioned, HDL is the "good" cholesterol—the kind you want more of. An HDL level of at least 60 milligrams per deciliter is desirable; lower than 35 mg/dL is too low. LDL, of course, is the "bad" cholesterol—the kind you want *less* of. An LDL level of less than 130 mg/dL is desirable; higher than 159 mg/dL is too high.

Total cholesterol is the third cholesterol reading that can help predict heart-disease risk. Actually, though, it's not so much an accurate predictor of risk as it is an accurate predictor of *non*risk. Anyone with a total cholesterol level of 150 mg/dL or lower is generally considered to be safe from heart disease. Note well, however, that risk of a heart attack doesn't reliably increase as total cholesterol increases. In fact, of Americans who have heart attacks, twice as many have total cholesterol levels between 150 and 200 mg/dL as have levels higher than 300 mg/dL.

Another useful indicator is the LDL/HDL ratio. Any ratio under 4 is considered health protective unless total cholesterol is above 300 mg/dL.

WHAT'S YOUR MAN'S RISK OF A FIRST HEART ATTACK?
To find out whether your partner's at higher than average risk of
a first heart attack compared to the general adult population, score
his risk factors on the lines below. (Check yourself, too!)

_____AGE: MEN

    0 points: Younger than 35

    1 point: 35 to 39

    2 points: 40 to 48

    3 points: 49 to 53

    4 points: 54+

_____AGE: WOMEN

    0 points: Younger than 42

    1 point: 42 to 44

    2 points: 45 to 54

    3 points: 55 to 73

    4 points 74+

_____FAMILY HISTORY

    2 points: My family has a history of heart disease or heart attacks
before age 60

_____INACTIVE LIFESTYLE

    1 point: I rarely exercise or do anything physically demanding

_____WEIGHT

    1 point: I'm more than 20 pounds over my ideal weight

_____SMOKING STATUS

    1 point: I'm a smoker

_____DIABETES

    1 point: I'm a male diabetic

    2 points: I'm a female diabetic

_____TOTAL CHOLESTEROL LEVEL

    0 points: Less than 240 mg/dL

    1 point: 240 to 315 mg/dL

    2 points: More than 315 mg/dL

_____HDL CHOLESTEROL LEVEL

0 points: 39 to 59 mg/dL

1 point: 30 to 38 mg/dL

2 points: Under 30 mg/dL

−1 point: Over 60 mg/dL

_____BLOOD PRESSURE

I don't take blood pressure medication; my blood pressure is (use your top or higher blood pressure number):

0 points: Less than 140 mm Hg

1 point: 140 to 170 mm Hg

2 points: Greater than 170 mm Hg

OR:

1 point: I'm currently taking blood pressure medication

_____**Total Points**

Scoring: If you scored 4 points or more, you could be at above average risk of a first heart attack compared to the general adult population. The more points you score, the greater your risk. If you have already had a heart attack or have heart disease, your heart attack risk is significantly higher. Only your doctor can evaluate your risk and recommend treatment plans to reduce your risk. If you don't know your cholesterol level or blood pressure, ask your doctor if your levels should be checked

Reprinted courtesy of Bristol-Myers Squibb Company

Tuberculosis Test

The tuberculin skin test with purified protein derivative (PPD) is used to tell whether a person has been infected with tuberculosis, a chronic bacterial infection. A positive PPD means that sometime in the past (and it could have been years earlier) the person was infected with the tuberculosis bacterium and developed antibodies (chemicals the body uses to fight off infection) specifically against TB. The disease can be spread when an infected person coughs or sneezes, spraying droplets containing the TB organism into the air. TB has become more common since the advent of AIDS because people whose immune systems are compromised are more susceptible to it.

The first stage of TB may produce no symptoms or symptoms similar to those of a common cold. In the second stage, symptoms might include a slight fever, night sweats, weight loss, and tiredness without obvious cause. Most commonly, TB affects the lungs, causing a cough, shortness of breath, and chest pain.

Often, TB doesn't progress past the first stage. The immune system resists the disease by destroying or walling off most of the bacteria in a fibrous capsule. However, in some cases, some of the bacteria remain alive and can reactivate the infection.

To test for the disease, a small amount of PPD is injected into the skin. If the injected area turns red and hard (this usually happens within 48 to 72 hours), the person is "PPD-positive," which indicates that he or she is carrying the antibody that's protective against the development of TB. In most cases, a positive test result simply means that the person has successfully fought the infection and won't get TB. Nevertheless, anyone with a positive PPD should be evaluated by a physician. Adults should be tested for TB antibody every five years.

Urine and Blood Tests

Part of most comprehensive physical exams, a routine urinalysis includes tests for glucose (sugar), protein, bilirubin and ketones. The presence of any of these substances in the urine usually indicates a health problem. Elevated glucose and ketones can be indicative of diabetes; elevated protein, of kidney problems, and elevated bilirubin, of liver disease. The urine sediment (the insoluble material that tends to sink to the bottom of the urine sample) also is examined under a microscope. Detection of debris or of white or red blood cells may indicate the presence of an infection, a tumor, or a disorder of the kidneys, bladder, or the tubes connecting them together and to the outside world (the ureter and the urethra, respectively).

Routine blood tests can alert doctors to the possible presence of a wide variety of conditions, including diabetes, liver disease, and kidney disease. The complete blood cell count (CBC) is the most common blood test. Each type of blood cell (white cells, red cells, and platelets) in a given volume of blood is counted. The results can indicate such problems as infections, leukemia, and various types of anemia, as well as other conditions. These tests should be done as frequently as preventive physical exams are recommended for any given age.

LOOK OUT FOR DASTARDLY DIABETES

Diabetes is one of the leading causes of death by disease in the U.S. In spite of that fact, about only half of the estimated 16 million Americans with diabetes realize that they have the disease. This ignorance is dangerous because the longer a person goes without treatment, the more damage is done to the blood vessels and organs, eventually leading to heart disease, stroke, nerve impairment, kidney disease or blindness. People with any of the following risk factors should be especially vigilant about being screened for diabetes:

- Obesity (more than 20 percent above ideal weight)
- Family history (parent or sibling with diabetes)

- Member of a high risk ethnic group (African American, Hispanic, Native American, Asian)
- Hypertension (blood pressure above 140/90 mm Hg)
- HDL cholesterol of 35 mg/dL or lower and/or a triglyceride level of 250 mg/dL or higher
- Abnormal results on an earlier glucose test

Source: American Diabetes Association

Electrocardiography

This test records the electrical forces produced during each heartbeat. It can help identify damage to the heart muscle, irregular heartbeat rhythms, enlargement of a chamber of the heart, or other damage caused by a heart attack. The test is painless and quick, and can be performed in a doctor's office. The patient lies on an examining table, undressed from the waist up. Electrodes are attached to the wrists, ankles, and chest. During the test patients should breathe normally but shouldn't move or talk, because any movement can distort the test results. Between the ages of 30 and 49, this test is recommended every three years for those who have high cholesterol or a family history of heart disease. The test is recommended every three years for *everyone* aged 50 or older.

Hemoccult

Hemoccult means hidden blood. In this simple test, designed to detect blood in the stool that isn't visible to the naked eye, a small amount of stool is put onto a plastic slide or specially treated paper. It's analyzed either in the doctor's office or at a laboratory. This test is recommended every year after the age of 50.

Sigmoidoscopy

During this procedure, the physician inserts a thin, lighted, tubular scope through the anus into the large bowel. The scope allows the doctor to examine visually the rectum and lower colon, where more than half of all large bowel cancers occur. The American Cancer Society recommends this test after the age of 50. If the first two annual tests are normal, the exam should be repeated every three to five years.

Overcoming an Aversion to Screening

It's important to discuss your partner's feelings about screening tests. They aren't preventive in the sense of stopping a disease before it has a chance to start, like quitting smoking does. But screening tests can detect diseases early, before they make a person feel ill or before a physician can identify them simply by taking a history and doing a physical exam. And in many cases, early intervention can prevent a bad outcome that might occur if treatment were delayed until the disease became clinically apparent.

However, many men—and women, too—have an understandable aversion to bad news. To avoid bad news about their health, they avoid doctors and screening tests. If your partner habitually avoids preventive health care, ask him why. Engage him in an open discussion about men and their attitudes toward preventive health care. Ask how he feels about the issues discussed in this chapter, including whether he would rather be treated for prostate cancer and live longer but with side effects, or preserve his short-term quality of life at the risk of dying younger.

With the help of your sensitive input, he may well realize that the inconveniences and indignities he fears aren't as important as protecting his health and his longevity. Point out that it's always better to know about a health problem than to have it catch you by surprise at a later stage, when treatment options are usually reduced. You also might point out that earlier treatment is often a lot less expensive, both in terms of direct costs and lost income, than later treatment.

Remind your man, too, that not every health problem requires invasive medical treatment. For example, if prostate-cancer screenings turn up a malignant tumor, watchful waiting—in which the tumor is evaluated periodically but no treatment is administered—is an option for some men, especially those who are older and have small, low-grade tumors that are unlikely to spread. Many other diseases and negative health conditions, such as high cholesterol, adult-onset diabetes, and hypertension, can be managed with lifestyle changes alone.

Most men adhere to maintenance recommendations for their cars because they know that doing so can increase a car's life and improve its overall functioning. If they notice a strange noise emanating from the engine, they have it checked out by a mechanic. Why? Because they know that to continue driving a vehicle that needs repairs may cause additional damage.

Point out to your partner that bringing his body to a medical office for the recommended screenings makes at least as much sense as bringing his car to a garage for an oil change and having the mechanic check the brakes, steering, fluid levels, electrical system, and engine-cooling system while it's there. In fact, it makes a heck of a lot more sense because, clearly, a man's life is more valuable than that of his car.

FIVE WAYS TO GET YOUR MAN TO THE DOCTOR
Need some ideas to help get your man to cross the threshold of
a physician's office? Try these:

1. Find a doctor who offers evening or Saturday appointments.
This will help you get around the number-one excuse offered by men who
avoid physicians: they're too busy at work to take time off for a doctor's
appointment. If your man says he doesn't have time on the weekends or
evenings either, ask him this: "Won't it take more time to recover from a
heart attack than it will to have your blood pressure and cholesterol checked
so that a heart attack might be avoided?"

**2. Help your partner get a recommendation for a primary care
doctor.** Ask the wives of his good friends which doctors their men
use. Although clinical qualifications are of primary importance, personality is also critical. Like any patient, your man needs to feel comfortable with his primary care physician in order to get the best care
possible. Chances are they'll be discussing some highly personal issues,
and feeling awkward with the doctor might lead your man to hold back
critical details.

3. Offer to go with your partner to an appointment. At the very
least, you can keep him company in the waiting room. If your partner wants,
you can be present at the end of the physical exam when the doctor discusses
his findings. When it comes to medical consultations, four ears are always
better than two.

**4. Call the doctor's office to ask exactly what tests and exams
are part of a complete physical for a man of your partner's age.**
(This can vary slightly by office.) Checking ahead will allow you to tell your
man exactly what to expect. It also will give him a chance to make a list of
questions based on the tests and exams that will be done (most of us find
it difficult to remember our questions as we sit naked and cold in a paper-
towel gown).

5. Ask for the medical history forms ahead of time. Usually, the receptionist in the doctor's office can mail you any history forms that your partner will be asked to fill out. He may feel more comfortable filling them out at home, where he can easily check dates or call a relative to ask questions about family history.

3

BOOST YOUR NUTRITION KNOWLEDGE

> *Real knowledge is to know the extent of one's ignorance.*
>
> *Confucius*

"I didn't know that fried calamari was bad for you," says Al Hodys, an attorney in Manhattan. "Debbie told me," he continues, referring to his wife, who is also an attorney. "I guess all fried foods are bad for you."

For a man like Al, whose father has had three angioplasties (the first at the age of 52), good nutrition needs to be based on more than guesswork. But even if your man has a squeaky-clean family history, his long-term health depends in large part on the food he feeds his body every day.

How does food affect health? A man who is overweight or doesn't eat a nutritionally sound diet is at increased risk of heart disease, stroke, diabetes, and several different cancers, including those of the colon, rectum, prostate, stomach, and esophagus. Hundreds of thousands of Americans die each year because they were either unhealthy eaters, obese, or both. In addition, many people lead lives that are hampered by chronic diseases

71

that might have been prevented if they had eaten a healthy diet.

Unfortunately, most men don't give nutrition a second thought. The statistics paint a troubling picture in which the average American man fails to meet even the most basic dietary recommendations. For example:

• Dietary guidelines issued by the U.S. Department of Agriculture (USDA), creators of the Food Guide Pyramid, recommend six to 11 servings of grain products per day. American men average just three.

• The daily recommendation for fruits and vegetables is five to nine servings. The average American adult barely manages to eat the minimum five—and that's counting the apples in apple pie, the lettuce and tomato on a Big Mac, the tomatoes in pizza sauce, and french fried potatoes.

• Of men aged 25 to 50, only 23 percent consume the previously recommended 800 milligrams (mg) of calcium daily. Now the Institute of Medicine recommends that men and women between the ages of 19 and 30 get 1,000 mg a day (about three-and-a-half servings of calcium-rich foods). Those older than 50 should get 1,200 mg per day. Obviously, even fewer than 23 percent of men meet the new, higher standard.

• The USDA recommends that fat make up no more than 30 percent of the energy (measured in calories) we get from food each day. However, many nutrition experts say a lower goal, such as 20 to 25 percent, would be healthier. No more than 10 percent of total calories should come from saturated fat, the type of fat that's most solid, and thus most dangerous to your health. How do American men stack up? On average, 33 percent of daily calories come from fat; 12 percent from saturated fat.

• The result of poor dietary habits is often excess weight. According to the most recent data from the Department of Health and Human Services, nearly one out of every three men between the ages of 20 and 74 tips the scales at a weight that's considered unhealthy (more than 20 percent above his medically recommended weight). That's up from 26 percent five years ago.

The human body uses the chemical compounds it extracts from food, including fats, sugars (carbohydrates), proteins, and vitamins, to function and to repair itself. Like most machines, it works better and lasts longer if you care for it properly and use the fuel recommended by the manufacturer. Obviously, unlike cars and lawn mowers, people don't come with instructions. Fortunately, scientists have been able to discover much about which substances in food are good or bad for the body. We human beings are busily writing our own care and maintenance manual.

This chapter presents a summary of some of the most important and widely accepted scientific advice about nutrition. We'll start by outlining the best nutrition strategy for your man and you. Then we'll describe 11 ways you can help your man improve his diet. Finally, we'll look at the role food plays in several common diseases. Along the way, you'll find inspiring stories of couples who have successfully changed their eating habits for the healthier.

A Nutrition Strategy for Your Man—and You

We strongly recommend that you and your partner aim to follow the recommendations in the Food Guide Pyramid, which was developed by the USDA and the U.S. Public Health Service. The pyramid was designed to help people choose foods that, eaten over the course of a day, add up to a well-balanced diet.

What is a well-balanced diet? The government has adopted the rule of thumb that to best promote health, about 60 percent of what we eat should be carbohydrates (starches and sugars found primarily in bread, rice, pasta, cereal, fruits, and vegetables); 30 percent (or less) should be fat, and 10 percent should be protein.

The Food Guide Pyramid translates that advice into the number of servings of different types of foods that we should eat in a given day. The pyramid represents a new way of thinking about food for most Americans. Many of us are used to planning meals around meat, then adding pasta, bread, or rice as a side dish. Too often, vegetables and fruits are little more than garnishes, if they appear at all.

To follow the advice in the Food Guide Pyramid, you'll need to plan meals around grain products, vegetables, and fruit, then use meat and other protein sources as side dishes. This may take a lot of mental readjustment—and a change in shopping habits as well—but the health benefits of such a diet will make the change worthwhile. (For tips on how to implement the pyramid guidelines in your home, see Chapter 4, "Create a Healthy Kitchen.")

Before we start our tour of the pyramid, we want to mention one major nutrient that doesn't appear there: water. Water plays an important role in nearly every major function that your body performs. It brings oxygen and nutrients to cells and removes wastes. It regulates body temperature, cushions joints, and helps to protect organs and tissues. Without it, we would live no more than a few days. (You can't say *that* about carbohydrates, protein, or fat.) Experts recommend drinking at least eight 8-ounce

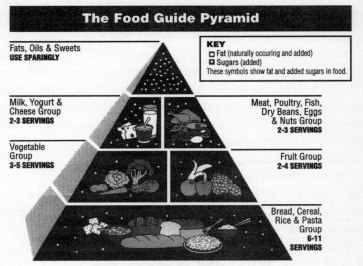

Source: U.S. Department of Agriculture,
and U.S. Department of Health and Human Services

glasses of water a day to keep your body hydrated and to help prevent kidney stones, fatigue, and constipation. Juices, milk and caffeine-free soft drinks can make up part of the eight-glasses-a-day requirement, but caffeine and alcohol actually contribute to dehydration.

Get in the habit of drinking water with meals and make it easy for your partner to drink water throughout the day by giving him a large plastic glass or sports bottle (emblazoned with the logo of his favorite team, perhaps) to keep at work.

Go for the Grains.

As you can see in the Food Guide Pyramid illustration, grain products are the foundation of a healthy diet. Six to 11 servings daily are recommended. A serving equals one slice of bread, an ounce of ready-to-eat cereal, or a half cup of cooked cereal, rice, or pasta.

Whether you should have six or 11 servings depends on your size and activity level. A small, inactive woman would need six servings a day. At the other end of the scale, a tall, large-framed, active man should aim for 11 servings.

Carbohydrates come in two basic varieties: simple (sugars) and complex (starches). Foods rich in starches are a better choice than foods rich in sugars because starches generally contain large amounts of minerals and vitamins, which sugars lack.

A diet rich in complex carbohydrates (such as whole-grain bread, pasta, rice, breakfast cereal, and starchy vegetables) has been shown to reduce the risk of heart disease and cancer.

Load Up on Fruits and Veggies.

Fruits and vegetables are the next step up in the pyramid. The recommendations call for three to five servings of vegetables and two to four of fruit daily. A serving equals a half cup cooked or chopped raw vegetables or fruit, one cup of raw leafy vegetables, three-quarters cup of vegetable or fruit juice, or one medium piece of whole fruit.

Because men generally consume more calories in a day than women, they should be eating at the upper end of the pyramid recommendations—eight or nine servings of fruits and vegetables per day. Most men (and women) don't even come close. In fact, the typical American diet is so devoid of fruits and vegetables that Paul Lachance, a Rutgers University nutritionist, summed up the situation like this: "Potatoes are this country's main source of vitamin C. Without french fries, we would have scurvy in America."

Eating lots of fresh fruits and vegetables will give your body the ammunition it needs to battle disease. Fruits and vegetables contain fiber, which protects against heart disease and cancers of the digestive tract and improves simple bowel function. Fruits and vegetables also contain vitamins and other substances that reduce risk of high blood pressure, heart disease, stroke, cancer, and diabetes.

In a study on diet and cancer risk at the University of California at Berkeley, researchers found that people who ate the most fruits and vegetables had half the cancer risk of people who ate the least. According to a study that followed 832 Massachusetts men for 20 years, for every three servings of fruits and vegetables a man eats daily, he reduces his risk of stroke by 22 percent.

Choose Protein Carefully.
Next up on the pyramid are the protein sources: milk and milk products (two to three servings daily), and meat, poultry, fish, eggs, beans, and nuts (two to three servings daily). Most Americans get twice as much protein as they need (men need about 63 grams; women need about 50 grams). While this extra protein may not pose a direct health threat, it certainly poses an indirect threat. The more protein you eat, the fewer grains, vegetables, and fruits you'll have room for. In addition, people who eat a lot of animal protein are swallowing a lot of fat and cholesterol, too.

Red meat is the largest source of saturated fat in the average American's diet. That means that frequent consumption increases risk of heart disease and stroke. In addition, men who eat red meat as a main dish five or more times a week are four times as likely to get colon cancer and twice as likely to get prostate cancer as men who rarely eat red meat.

Experts recommend no more than three servings a week of red meat. Bear in mind that the size of a meat serving is smaller than many people think: 2 to 3 ounces (about the size of a deck of cards).

As you try to convince your man to eat less red meat, remember that he may be more attached to the stuff than you are. Researchers at the University of Michigan found that while women crave foods like chocolate, cakes, pastries, and ice cream, men crave steaks, roasts, hamburgers, sausage, and pizza. Denying a craving completely usually results in overindulgence once you give in to the craving. For that reason, it may be best to cut back on red meat (eat it less often and reduce the size of a portion) instead of trying to eliminate it.

There may be more to a man's attachment to beef than cravings. In our culture, eating red meat projects an image that's strong, rugged, and masculine. Take, for example, a nutrition column that appeared in *Men's Health* magazine in the July/August 1996 issue. It will give you an idea of what you may be up against. The column offered low-fat versions of "manly foods" such as chili, sloppy joes, and hamburgers. It was titled, "Macho, Macho meals" and carried a subsidiary headline that read: "Want to lower your cholesterol without wimpifying your diet? Here are 27 cool, manly foods that help your heart."

The message for you: Your time might be better spent learning how to reduce the fat in his favorite meals than it would be trying to convince him to eat veggieburgers.

Keep a Tight Rein on Fat.

Topping off the pyramid are fats, oils, and sweets, which should be used sparingly. Nutrition experts recommend that we keep dietary cholesterol to less than 300 milligrams daily and fat to less than 30 percent of daily calories.

For Americans, this is a difficult task. The foods many

of us grew up with are high in fat: hamburgers, hot dogs, fried chicken, steak, macaroni and cheese, ham and cheese sandwiches, bacon and eggs, and so on. If the foods themselves aren't fatty (vegetables, potatoes), we often make them so by slathering on butter or sour cream. If your man grew up that way, chances are good that he favors those high-fat foods and will be reluctant to give them up. He may associate them with feelings of comfort and security.

Try to establish new rituals to replace the old. Instead of bacon and eggs every day, have them on Sundays only. Use low-fat ground turkey breast instead of ground beef to make burgers, meatballs, and meat loaf. Instead of a ham sandwich with mayonnaise, try turkey breast with mustard. These changes may seem unnatural at first, but with time your man's personal taste will change and he'll look forward to the new family favorites as much as he did the old. For more ideas on healthy food substitutions, see Chapter 4, "Create a Healthy Kitchen."

 HOW BIG IS A SERVING?
So you know you're supposed to encourage your partner to eat fewer servings of meat and more servings of fruits and vegetables. But what constitutes a portion?

FRUITS
1 medium apple, banana, orange
½ cup of chopped, cooked, or canned fruit
¾ cup of fruit juice

VEGETABLES
1 cup of raw leafy vegetables
½ cup of other cooked or chopped raw vegetables
¾ cup vegetable juice

GRAINS

1 slice bread
1 ounce ready-to-eat cereal
½ cup of cooked cereal, rice, pasta

BEANS AND NUTS

½ cup cooked dry beans
2 tablespoons peanut butter
⅓ cup nuts

DAIRY FOODS AND EGGS

1 cup milk or yogurt
1½ ounces of natural cheese
2 ounces processed cheese
1 egg

MEATS

2–3 ounces of cooked lean meat, poultry, fish

Source: U.S. Department of Agriculture and U.S. Department of Health and Human Services: *Nutrition and Your Health: Dietary Guidelines for Americans*

Social Eating Can Be Healthy Eating

According to a study at Duke University, men are most at risk of overeating when they're happy, excited, or out socializing with the guys. Al Hodys, the 35-year-old reformed calamari eater we introduced at the beginning of this chapter, is a case in point. Al used to spend a lot of time eating out with male friends—a ritual that frequently involved buckets of chicken wings and big steaks. "Meat is macho," says Al. "Fruit is not. Fruit salad is just not something you're going to order when you're out with the guys."

When pressed further, he explains that a lot of men—

especially younger men—resent the pressure in our increasingly health-conscious society to avoid high-fat favorites. When men sit down at a restaurant table together, says Al, the subconscious thinking goes something like this: "Let's face it. We all like steak. I'm not going to give in to our society's pervasive fear of fat. I'm strong enough to sit down and have a steak with my friends without having to worry about my health." Giving in to the fear of fat would be "wimpy." It would admit vulnerability, which most men don't like to do because they equate vulnerability with weakness.

Your partner's health won't suffer if he eats a baconburger and french fries when he's out with the guys—as long as he doesn't do it every week, and as long as he makes healthy food choices when he's at home or at work.

What can you do if your partner socializes a lot? Help him become aware of situations—like watching the game with friends—in which he eats unhealthy foods. Being aware of a habit or pattern of behavior is the first step toward changing it. He may choose to avoid situations and events that lead him to eat high-fat foods. However, a more realistic strategy might be to go to such events less frequently or to learn how to make healthier food choices in social situations.

You might suggest that your partner eat a healthy snack before going out. If he's feeling full, he'll be less inclined to camp in front of the potato chips. When he's out for dinner with friends, he can eat smaller portions of what everyone else is eating—no one will notice. For example he can order the 10-ounce sirloin instead of the 16-ounce and he can eat half of the french fries on his plate.

Introduce your partner to the concept of food substitution, one of the most important ways to change permanently, over time, from a less healthy to a more healthy eating pattern. For example, when he's out, your partner can order tortilla chips and salsa instead of nachos with cheese and ground beef. He can have pie for dessert but skip the ice cream. He can have steak, but a lean cut like flank, club, tenderloin, sirloin, or London broil instead of prime rib, T-bone or rib-eye. He can have a hamburger, but order it medium or well done (the extra time on the grill eliminates some fat). He can have a baked potato instead of french fries, with margarine instead of sour cream or butter.

Aside from providing these practical suggestions, you can try to change your partner's mind about what constitutes "manly" eating. Isn't choosing healthy foods more manly than bowing to peer pressure to order prime rib with french fries or a pepperoni pizza with extra cheese? Tell your man that eating healthy is a sign of intelligence and strength because it takes thought and will power to do so.

Make Variety Your Man's Mantra

A word of caution: Don't zero in on any one vitamin, mineral, phytochemical (chemical compound found in food), or food as a shield against disease. The key, experts agree, is to include all of the foods that contain beneficial compounds. That means eating lots of a variety of fruits, vegetables, beans, grains, and low-fat dairy products.

You've probably heard of the French paradox—the relatively low incidence of heart disease among the French in spite of their typically high-fat diets. Scientists have long tried to identify one magic bullet—garlic or red wine, for example—that could account for this puzzle. One recent study points to the *variety* of foods consumed by the French, rather than to one particular food, as a possible answer. In a survey of more than 800 men and women living near Paris, researchers found that 90 percent of participants ate from all five food groups—dairy, meats, grains, fruits, and vegetables—daily. In contrast, only about 33 percent of Americans eat from all five food groups daily.

What's Weight Got to Do With It?

When it comes to avoiding disease, healthy eating should be coupled with healthy weight. Why? Because obesity is the second leading preventable cause of death in the U.S., leading to some 300,000 deaths annually. Obese men are more likely to have (get ready, it's a long list): heart disease, stroke, diabetes, prostate cancer, colon cancer, high blood pressure, high cholesterol, gallstones, gout, osteoarthritis, back pain, and varicose veins.

According to the government's National Health and Nutrition Examination Survey, Americans are getting fatter. Today, 59 percent of American men (and 49 percent of women) weigh more than is considered healthy for their height. Ten years ago, 51 percent of men (and 41 percent of women) weighed in above the healthy range for their height.

Assessing Weight and Body Shape

How do you know if your man's weight is healthy? The best way to determine that is to calculate his body-mass index (BMI), a scientific measure of each person's height-weight relationship. The higher the number, the less healthy a BMI the person has. Thus, a BMI of 19 to 24 is considered healthy; 25 to 27, overweight; and 28 or more, obese.

	Healthy Weight						Overweight			Obese	
BMI	**19**	**20**	**21**	**22**	**23**	**24**	**25**	**26**	**27**	**28**	**29**
5'5"	114	120	126	132	138	144	150	156	162	168	174
5'6"	118	124	130	136	142	148	155	161	167	173	179
5'7"	121	127	134	140	146	153	159	166	172	178	185
5'8"	125	131	138	144	151	158	164	171	177	184	190
5'9"	128	135	142	149	155	162	169	176	182	189	196
5'10"	132	139	146	153	160	167	174	181	188	195	202
5'11"	136	143	150	157	165	172	179	186	193	200	208
6'	140	147	154	162	169	177	184	191	199	206	213
6'1"	144	151	159	166	174	182	189	197	204	212	219
6'2"	148	155	163	171	179	186	194	202	210	218	225
6'3"	152	160	168	176	184	192	200	208	216	224	232
6'4"	156	164	172	180	189	197	205	213	221	230	238

If the weight you're looking for isn't in the table, you can calculate BMI by following these simple steps:

1. Multiply your partner's weight in pounds by 705.
2. Divide the result by your partner's height in inches.
3. Divide again by your partner's height in inches.

BMI is a good measure of health, but it's not perfect. A bodybuilder whose weight is mostly muscle may have a high BMI, but he probably isn't fat. In addition, the location of body fat can make a difference. Excess weight that's carried around the hips and thighs (a "pear" shape) is less of a health threat than excess weight carried around the abdomen (an "apple" shape). An apple shape is tied to a higher risk of heart disease, stroke, and diabetes than is a pear shape.

With your partner's permission, you can determine whether his weight is dangerously distributed by calculating his waist-to-hip ratio. Here's how:

1. Using a tape measure, find the circumference of his waist at its narrowest point. (Your partner's stomach muscles should be relaxed.)

2. Measure the circumference of his hips at the widest point (where his buttocks protrude most).

3. Divide the waist measurement by the hip measurement to determine his waist-to-hip ratio. For men, a ratio of less than 0.95 is recommended. (For women, it's 0.8 or less.)

If your partner's BMI indicates that he's overweight, or if his waist-to-hip ratio indicates that he not only has too much fat, but also that it's in the wrong place, what can you do about it? If he's ready to change his eating habits, you can share what you've learned in this chapter with him. Then you can use the information and advice in Chapter 4, "Create a Healthy Kitchen," to put theory into practice. Remember, your goal should be to help your partner change his eating habits permanently, not just to help him restrict calories temporarily so that he can drop a few pounds fast.

Weight Loss Made Simple

The focus of any weight-loss effort should be on eating healthy foods, exercising (see Chapter 5, "Get Your Man Moving"), and keeping calorie intake in check. Although we're not suggesting that your partner become a strict calorie counter, he may find it useful to keep track for a couple of days. Then if his goal is to maintain his current weight, he can measure his average day's total caloric intake against the number of calories he should be consuming. If he wants to lose weight, he can calculate the number of calories he would have to consume to maintain the lower weight, and gradually reduce his intake to that level. **Here's how your partner can calculate the number of calories he should eat in a day.**

• If your partner's practically sedentary or a sometime-exerciser, he should multiply his weight by 12. For example, if he weighs 180 (and that's a healthy weight for him), he could eat 2,160 calories (180 times 12) and still maintain his weight. If your partner's overweight he can find his target caloric intake by multiplying his target weight by 12. For example, if he wants to weigh 160 pounds, he would multiply 160 by 12 (1,920 calories).

• If your partner's moderately active (a half-hour of steady aerobic work, three to six times a week), multiply weight by 15.

• If your partner's very active (an hour or more a day of vigorous activity), multiply weight by 18.

HOW MUCH FAT SHOULD YOUR MAN EAT?
It's widely agreed that no one should get more than 30 percent of total daily calories from fat. However, many experts urge us to eat even less than that. Use the following table to see if your partner's on track. (To find out how many calories your man should consume in a day, see the above bulleted list.)

Calorie Intake	30% Fat Diet	25% Fat Diet	20% Fat Diet
1,800	60 grams	50 grams	40 grams
1,900	63 grams	53 grams	42 grams
2,000	67 grams	56 grams	44 grams
2,100	70 grams	58 grams	47 grams
2,200	73 grams	61 grams	49 grams
2,300	77 grams	64 grams	51 grams
2,400	80 grams	67 grams	53 grams
2,500	83 grams	69 grams	56 grams
2,600	87 grams	72 grams	58 grams
2,700	90 grams	75 grams	60 grams

If your partner is ready to lose weight, the first step is for him to set a realistic goal. Many weight-loss experts agree that trying to lose 10 percent of total body weight is an attainable goal that will provide some health benefits for anyone who's overweight. Once your partner has lost 10 percent of his weight and kept it off for six months, if he's still plumper than he would like to be, he may want to set another goal: to lose 10 percent of his new weight.

Eleven Ways to Help Your Man Eat Healthy

As we described in Chapter 1 of this book, there are certain motivational stages people go through on their way to making a lifestyle change. Use the information and tips in that chapter to determine which stage your partner has reached and to help bump him up to the next stage.

Although you can't change your man's habits for him, you *can* create an atmosphere that fosters change. Here's how:

1. Be positive. Negative comments will get you no-where fast. Instead of chastising your partner because he isn't ready to give up bacon, find something to praise him about. Maybe he loves pasta. Point out that pasta is part of a healthy diet. Perhaps he always has a glass of orange juice in the morning. You might say: "You're so good about having juice every morning. I'm going to try to do the same more consistently than I have been."

Once you've shown a willingness to improve your own eating habits and have pointed out the positive aspects of your partner's diet, you'll be in a much better position to say: "I'll bet that *when you're ready*, you'll be able to cut back on bacon, too."

2. If you're the cook in the family, follow the Food Guide Pyramid guidelines when preparing a meal. This may mean changing the way you think about meals. Train yourself to think of meat as a side dish by asking your partner whether he feels like having rice, potatoes, or pasta tonight instead of asking whether he'd like beef or chicken. Begin serving smaller portions of meat and larger portions of the healthier foods you used to think of as side dishes (rice, pasta, vegetables, salad).

3. Make sure your partner is a willing accomplice. If you start serving tofu and couscous without his agreeing to try those things, you're likely to encounter a negative response. For example, you may be tempted to use a low-fat meat alternative next time you make chili—just to see if your partner notices. Chances are that he *will* notice (meat substitutes, while enjoyed by many, don't taste exactly like ground beef).

If your partner has already decided he wants to eat less meat, he may get a kick out of your little experiment. On the other hand, if he's on the fence about the whole idea of changing the way he eats, a prank like this could really turn him off. Instead, you could ask him: "How would you like to try using low-fat cheese on our pizza one time to see if we like it?" Or: "You know, I'd like to try making an omelet with an egg substitute. How do you feel about that?"

The bottom line is that sly changes send this message: "*I'm* going to change *your* eating habits," which, of course, is impossible. The decision to make a change—even a small one—has to come from the person doing the changing. Your goal is to build a partnership, and trust—not trickery—builds partnerships. Use what you've learned about nutrition to convince your partner that the changes you're proposing are worth making.

4. Whenever possible, point out a tangible benefit when suggesting a change. For example, next time you and your partner eat baked potatoes, ask him to try topping his with five squirts of a spray margarine substitute instead of a tablespoon of the real stuff. Tell him he'll save 11 grams of fat if he does. That's the amount of fat in a 3-ounce flank steak—wouldn't he rather have the steak? Even if the spray doesn't taste as good as the margarine, he may think the sacrifice is worth making when you frame it this way.

5. Don't be shy about using sex as a motivational tool. Take a lesson from *Men's Health* magazine, which has been offering health and fitness advice to men for 11 years. An article in the October 1997 issue tells readers: "The fact is, men who live a healthy lifestyle drive women wild, and that's as good a reason as any to stay fit. . . . So when you're feeling unmotivated, ponder the big prize: sex."

Let your partner know that his efforts to live a healthier lifestyle drive you wild. Tell him he looks sexy perusing produce in the supermarket and that you think it's fetching when he orders fish.

Some men think it's unmanly to take care of themselves; they're under the impression that real men don't need maintenance. Make sure your man knows that while you already find him sexy, it turns you on to see him working to maintain or improve his health and well-being.

6. Go easy on the empathy. In general, researchers have found that when a woman wants to help someone, she offers empathy and support. Men, on the other hand, offer information and/or solutions. Because people tend to offer others what they themselves would want in a given situation, we can assume that men find information more useful than empathy. If a man is looking for facts and/or a solution, he may find it frustrating to be told over and over again, "I understand what you're going through."

For example, a woman trying to encourage a man to reduce his fat intake might say, "I know how hard it must be for you to give up the foods you're used to eating, but we really need to cut fat from our diet. Let's both try to make better choices." That type of statement doesn't help a man do what he needs to do: make logical decisions and settle on a course of action that will solve his problem.

What he wants more than empathy is information. So a woman might have more success with a statement like this: "Eating a hamburger puts 16 grams of fat into your body. Adding 3 ounces of bacon increases the total fat by 42 grams. How about trying a burger without bacon?"

7. Tread softly around your man's ego. Having said that men want information, we need to point out that information has to be offered carefully. In her book *You Just Don't Understand*, Deborah Tannen writes that "giving information frames one as the expert, superior in knowledge, and the other as uninformed, inferior in knowledge. . . ." She goes on to explain that because appearing informed and self-sufficient is important to men, some "resist receiving information from others, especially women." This trait may annoy you, but if you want to improve your partner's diet, you'll have to accept and try to work around it.

How can you phrase advice so that it's palatable to your partner? First, as discussed earlier, don't tell your partner what to do. Next, ask yourself whether your partner will perceive what you're about to say as sharing information or nagging. If you've already told him that the cheese he puts in his scrambled eggs adds a lot of fat, don't mention it again. He's not continuing to use cheese because he has forgotten what you said. He's doing so because he's not ready to give it up. Instead, try giving him another option: he could make his scrambled eggs healthier without giving up cheese by using an egg substitute and adding vegetables.

Debbie has greatly improved the quality of Al's diet. What's the secret of her success? "She's very conscious about not nagging," says Al. "She doesn't want to fall into a relationship pattern where she nags and I resist. So she chooses her spots."

If your man resists receiving nutrition advice from you, try an indirect approach. For example, subscribe to a men's magazine that features nutrition articles. Editors of publications intended for men have a knack for presenting information in a humorous, chummy way that may be easier for your man to accept than your own words of wisdom. In addition, such publications will give *you* information— like nutrition news, healthy recipes, and exercise tips (not to mention interesting insights into the minds of men)— that you can use.

8. Never say "don't". No one likes to be told what to do, so stay away from statements beginning with the word don't, as in: "Don't eat that cake." Adam and Eve didn't take well to dietary orders ("Don't eat the apple"), and neither will your partner.

"Men don't like mandates," says Michael Lafavore, editor-in-chief of *Men's Health* magazine. "They won't do something simply because someone tells them they should. Men like choices. They want to know: What are the choices and what are the pros and cons of each choice? The best approach is to say: 'Here are the consequences; here are your options. You decide.'"

That's just what Debbie does when she sees Al make an unhealthy choice. She selects her words carefully to avoid sounding as though she's telling him what he should and shouldn't eat. Instead, she presents Al with the information he seems to be lacking, then moves on to another topic, leaving the decision up to him.

For example, one day they were in a restaurant and Al, thinking he was making a healthy selection, said he was going to order a tuna-salad sandwich. "Have it if you want," said Debbie, "but realize that tuna salad isn't as healthy as you think. The mayonnaise is loaded with fat."

When Debbie introduced Al to Special K cereal, he loved it. He thought he was having a spectacularly healthy breakfast. But Debbie noticed he was having trouble with portion control. "I was making gargantuan bowls—after three of *my* servings, the box would be gone," says Al. "Debbie showed me on the box where it says how big a serving is." Again, Debbie simply gave Al the information he needed to make a better decision for himself.

9. Start small. Start with small changes—like trying meatballs made of low-fat turkey breast instead of ground beef, or using 1-percent milk instead of whole milk or 2-percent—before tackling big changes like eating some meat-free meals. Remember that gradual change leads to permanent changes.

Simple changes that Al has made to his diet since meeting Debbie include passing on rolls before dinner; using low-fat cream cheese on bagels; using romaine lettuce instead of iceberg (romaine has more nutrients); ordering a salad with a light dressing on the side instead of a Caesar salad; avoiding anything in an alfredo sauce; substituting "no-cheese" pizza for the regular kind; and avoiding fried foods.

Having successfully reduced the fat content of his diet, Al's next goal is to start eating more fruits and vegetables. To improve your chances of meeting a broad goal like "eating more fruits and vegetables," break it into a series of concrete "mini" goals. For example, you and your partner might start by eating a piece of fruit with lunch three days a week, then five days a week, then every day. Once that becomes a habit, try adding a serving of vegetables to dinner by making salad a routine part of your evening meal or by snacking on carrot and celery sticks as you cook.

10. Suggest and institute changes one at a time. The more changes you and your partner take on at once, the less likely you are to succeed at any of them. Why? Contrary to popular belief, people don't have bottomless wells of willpower. Researchers have found that people stick with a demanding task, such as solving complex math problems, for a shorter time if they have to simultaneously use their willpower to resist a temptation like fresh-baked cookies. The lesson is to discourage your partner from trying to overhaul his diet, quit smoking, and start an exercise program all at once.

11. Practice what you preach. The best way to encourage your partner to adopt healthier eating habits is to do so yourself. Researchers in Britain found that, over the course of a year, men who showed the largest reductions in heart-disease risk factors (including BMI, blood pressure, cholesterol levels, and glucose levels) had partners who showed similar improvements. The researchers believe that partners help to reinforce each other's lifestyle changes.

That means that if he's giving up ice cream, you have to give up ice cream—or at least refrain from having it in the house and from eating it in front of him. If you start eating fruit on your cereal and making a habit of drinking orange juice with breakfast (two servings of fruit down for the day), he's more likely to engage in the same behavior.

Leading by Example

Often, men are inspired to make healthy changes by the women they love. When Sheila Beahm, a 35-year-old commercial airline pilot in Hawaii, met Larry Schuermann, a 39-year-old builder in the Lake Tahoe area, he was carrying an extra 20 pounds despite his active lifestyle.

"The extra weight bothered Larry," says Sheila, "but he was resigned to it. He didn't realize he could lose it by making a few simple changes to his diet. He was clueless about the idea of a balanced meal. He was eating a lot of cookies, cheese, and fast food."

Sheila explained the perils of fat to Larry and pointed out which foods in his diet were responsible for his weight gain. However, she didn't pressure Larry to adopt her healthy eating habits. Her patience was soon rewarded.

"He learned a lot just from watching what I eat," says Sheila. "I eat a lot of plain rice. So I bought him a rice cooker. When he started eating rice, he'd cover it in butter and salt. Now he eats it plain and loves it. In fact, every time we go to a wedding he buys a rice cooker as a gift."

Fish gradually replaced meat in Larry's diet. Skim milk replaced whole. He made that change by working gradually from 2-percent milk, to 1-percent, to skim. He uses only low-fat cheese. "Larry couldn't believe that in three months he was 20 pounds lighter," says Sheila. "He lost the weight without ever feeling like he was dieting."

Larry credits Sheila with being a good role model and a good source of information. He says that he feels more energetic and that he no longer gets the low back pain he used to experience periodically. Last, but not necessarily least: "Clothes that had stopped fitting fit again," says Larry.

Roman LePree, a 24-year-old magician living in Myrtle Beach, South Carolina, was similarly inspired by his 22-year-old fiancée, Michelle Bromley. When Michelle lost 50 pounds with the help of a weight-loss center, Roman decided to follow suit. He lost 40 pounds. Both have kept the lost weight off for three years by permanently changing their eating habits and making a commitment to exercise.

"I think he decided to lose weight when he saw how much better I looked and felt," says Michelle. "Once he changed his habits, it was easier for me to maintain my weight loss. It helps to have someone right next to you doing the same thing."

In the beginning, Roman had a lot to learn. "At first, he'd say: 'You tell me what I can eat, and I'll eat it,' " says Michelle.

Changing Habits

The couple points out that changing their recreational habits has helped them maintain their weight loss. "It used to be that everything we did was centered around food," says Michelle. The couple would go out for dinner and a movie—with candy. Or they would order pizza or cook some macaroni and cheese to eat while watching a video at home.

"One of the reasons I don't watch movies much anymore is because doing so makes me want to eat when I shouldn't be eating," says Michelle. Today, a typical date for the couple is more likely to involve a game of racquetball or beach volleyball.

One way Michelle helps Roman is by packing his lunch. It always consists of fruit, a vegetable, and a sandwich. Low-fat Twinkies are an occasional treat. For days when Roman has to eat out, Michelle did some research. "I've told Roman the lowest fat foods to get at every fast-food restaurant," says Michelle. (We'll give you tips for eating out in Chapter 4, "Create a Healthy Kitchen.")

As you can see from this chapter, there are many ways to help your man eat healthier—without nagging. If your partner is ready for change, use a blend of our tips and your own ideas to develop an approach that suits his style.

Debbie Bigel has managed to do so quite successfully. Since meeting her, Al has lost six of the 12 pounds he had put on after a back injury kept him from exercising. "I feel great," he says, giving Debbie her full share of credit. "She doesn't force changes on me; she educates me."

Education is, indeed, an important tool for a woman who wants to help her man get healthy. As mentioned earlier, the first instinct of a man faced with a problem is to gather the information he needs to settle on a logical course of action. The rest of this chapter is devoted to giving you the information you'll need to sell your partner on the health benefits of a healthy diet.

Using Food to Fight Cardiovascular Disease

Each year cardiovascular diseases (CVD)—including coronary heart disease, stroke, and hypertension (high blood pressure)—are responsible for about 460,000 deaths among American men and 500,000 deaths among American women. Note that more women than men die of cardiovascular diseases each year. If you're one of the many women who think they're not at risk for CVD, bear this statistic in mind: One in two women will eventually die of heart disease or stroke; one in 25 women will eventually die of breast cancer. We point this out to emphasize that it's important for women to join their partners in the effort to reduce personal risk factors for cardiovascular disease.

Although some risk factors for CVD run in families, diet and other lifestyle choices can determine whether family tendencies are played out. For those who already have CVD, dietary changes can help keep the use of medications and surgical procedures to a minimum. In some cases, lifestyle changes can actually reverse the progress of cardiovascular disease.

Be aware that heart attacks and strokes can occur without warning. Forty-eight percent of men (and 63 percent of women) who die suddenly of coronary heart disease had no prior symptoms of CVD. So don't let your partner lull himself into a state of inertia simply because he feels fine.

Heart attacks and strokes (sometimes called brain attacks) usually stem from a condition called atherosclerosis, which occurs when a hard material called plaque builds up on the inner walls of the arteries. Plaque is made up of cholesterol, scar tissue, calcium, and other substances. Plaque buildup can occur when a person consumes too much dietary fat and cholesterol. The problem is compounded when he or she eats too little fiber and too few fruits and vegetables.

Understanding Cholesterol

Despite its reputation as a clogger of arteries, cholesterol isn't all bad. The body needs cholesterol to carry out essential functions like repairing cell walls and producing internal "messenger" chemicals called hormones. Here's the catch: The body makes all the cholesterol it needs; any cholesterol you add via food is excess cholesterol.

To make things interesting, there are two types of cholesterol, commonly referred to as good cholesterol and bad cholesterol. This distinction doesn't exist in food, it only comes into play in your body. Both types of cholesterol are carried in your bloodstream by molecules called lipoproteins. Low-density lipoproteins (LDLs) are the bad guys—they clog arteries. High-density lipoproteins (HDLs) are the good guys—they help rid the body of excess LDLs. Like the world in general, your bloodstream needs fewer bad guys and more good guys. As you'll see, in your bloodstream at least, there are ways to reduce the number of bad guys and increase the number of good guys.

When doctors talk about a cholesterol profile, they're referring to the measurement of three aspects of cholesterol: LDLs, HDLs, and total cholesterol (the sum of the first two). Experts define a desirable total cholesterol level as below 200 mg/dL (milligrams of cholesterol per deciliter of blood). But a man who meets that criteria may still be at increased risk for heart disease if his HDL count is low (35 mg/dL or below). Conversely, a high total cholesterol count is less cause for concern in a man who has a high level of HDL cholesterol (60 mg/dL or more).

You and your partner can reduce LDL cholesterol in the blood by avoiding dietary cholesterol and saturated fat. Many people are surprised to learn that it's actually more important to avoid saturated fat than cholesterol. Why? Because saturated fat stimulates the body to produce more LDL cholesterol.

In addition to eating fewer foods that are high in fat and cholesterol, you and your partner can improve your cholesterol profiles by eating more foods high in soluble fiber (apples, oranges, grapefruits, oat and wheat bran cereals, beans), and foods rich in the chemical compounds called phytochemicals (garlic, leeks, onions, green tea, red grapes, soybeans).

HDL cholesterol can be increased, primarily through exercise. Smokers can increase their HDLs by quitting. Some studies suggest that eating smaller meals throughout the day raises HDL cholesterol and lowers total cholesterol. Losing weight is another way to improve your cholesterol profile.

FABULOUS FIBER!

There are two kinds of fiber: soluble, which dissolves in the digestive system, and insoluble, which doesn't. Soluble fiber helps to prevent heart disease and stroke by lowering cholesterol. It also helps to prevent diabetes by moderating blood glucose levels, and is thought to play a role in slowing the growth of cancer in the breast and prostate.

Insoluble fiber helps to reduce risk of constipation, hemorrhoids, diverticulosis, irritable colon, and colon cancer.

How much fiber should we eat? Experts recommend at least 20 to 30 grams daily—about twice as much as the average American consumes. Most fruits and vegetables contain a mixture of soluble and insoluble fiber, with one or the other predominating. Foods that are good sources of soluble fiber include legumes (dried beans, peas, peanuts, lentils), fruits (particularly apples and oranges), bran, barley, and oats. Good sources of insoluble fiber include nuts, seeds, brown rice, whole-grain cereals and breads, legumes, unpeeled vegetables, fruits, and wheat bran.

Blood-Pressure Basics

High blood pressure, another important risk factor for heart disease and stroke, can be aggravated by high cholesterol levels in the blood. When cholesterol deposits (plaque) form at points inside the arterial walls, it becomes more difficult for blood to pass through the arteries.

As a result, the body increases blood pressure to help blood get where it needs to go. With blood flowing at increased force, the inner walls of the arteries are more prone to damage. Plaque sticks to the damaged spots on arterial walls like Play-Doh sticks to your carpet. And so high cholesterol and high blood pressure continue to aggravate each other.

For the roughly 50 million Americans who have hypertension, reducing blood pressure is of vital importance. Why? Hypertension increases a person's risk of heart disease and stroke—the first and third most common causes of death in the nation. It also increases risk of kidney damage and vision loss. One study by the National Institutes on Aging found that high blood pressure may actually shrink parts of the brain. The researchers found that people with hypertension were more likely to have significantly smaller brain size and poorer verbal memory and language-comprehension skills than people of the same age who had normal blood pressure.

In most cases, doctors don't know what causes hypertension, although it can be brought on by certain treatable illnesses, such as hypothyroidism. If that's the case, which it is less than 5 percent of the time, blood pressure usually returns to normal once the underlying illness is successfully treated.

Although a few researchers dispute the importance of reducing salt intake to maintain a healthy blood pressure, most experts still advise cutting back. And all agree that reducing salt intake is essential for people who have hypertension.

Most of us get far more than the recommended daily intake of 2,400 milligrams of sodium. American men consume an estimated 4,000 milligrams per day; women an estimated 3,000 milligrams. Many people are surprised to learn that adding salt during cooking and at the table aren't the prime culprits. They account for only 15 percent of the salt we consume. Salt that occurs naturally in food accounts for another 10 percent. The remaining 75 percent of salt we consume comes from processed foods.

Reducing salt intake isn't the only way to reduce blood pressure. Other ways include exercising; maintaining a healthy weight; not smoking; managing stress effectively; and not overindulging in alcoholic beverages (more than two drinks a day can raise your blood pressure; three can cause hypertension).

Adequate consumption of certain nutrients is associated with reduced risk of hypertension. One notable study on nutrition and blood pressure has been dubbed the DASH (Dietary Approaches to Stop Hypertension) diet. Some of the 459 adults studied had blood pressure that was considered at the high end of normal; others had hypertension.

In the study, conducted at five medical centers across the country, patients were divided into three groups. The first ate a typical American diet—low in fruits and vegetables and high in fats. Patients in the second group were given extra fruits and vegetables, but were allowed to eat the same amount of fat as the first group. The third group ate a low fat diet (25 percent of calories from fat) that included nine to 10 servings of fruits and vegetables a day, along with low-fat milk and yogurt. The fruits and vegetables made the diet rich in potassium; the milk products contributed calcium and magnesium. All three minerals are thought to play a role in moderating blood pressure.

For subjects in the third group, blood pressure was reduced significantly both among those who at the outset had a slightly elevated pressure and those with true hypertension. Those with hypertension saw the biggest average improvement: an 11.4-point reduction in systolic pressure and a 5.5-point decrease in diastolic pressure. For those with slightly elevated (but still considered normal) blood pressure, systolic pressure dropped an average of 3.5 points and diastolic pressure dropped an average of 2.1 points.

The study indicates that a diet high in fruits and vegetables and low in fat can help prevent hypertension in those at risk. It also indicates that some people who already have hypertension may be able to avoid a lifetime of medication—or to get by with less medication—by altering their diets. That's important because, like any medication, drugs used to lower blood pressure can cause undesirable side effects. However, no one should stop taking blood pressure medication without first consulting his or her physician.

WHY YOUR MAN NEEDS CALCIUM

Usually, it's women who are being urged to get enough calcium to protect themselves from osteoporosis, the bone-thinning disease. But men need the protection offered by calcium, too. Although most common in women, one and a half million men in this country have osteoporosis. Some 3.5 million more are at high risk of developing it. In fact, American men age 50 or older have a greater chance of suffering an osteoporosis-related fracture than of developing prostate cancer.

Men most at risk for osteoporosis include those who are of European descent; eat a poor diet; smoke; take steroids; habitually take aluminum-containing antacids (such as Maalox or Mylanta); have a chronically low level of testosterone (impotence may be a sign of this); or have a family history of osteoporosis.

In addition to reducing risk of osteoporosis, studies have shown that calcium may reduce risk of hypertension. The mineral also may play a role in some cancers—population studies have linked low levels of calcium to high rates of colon and breast cancer.

Most men don't consume the recommended amount of calcium (1,000 mg daily for men 50 and younger; 1,200 mg for those older than 50). Calcium-rich foods include milk and milk products such as yogurt, cheese, and ice cream. (Of course, it's important to choose low-fat versions of these foods.) Calcium is also present in some green vegetables (including broccoli and string beans), some seafood (including shrimp and canned salmon), and soybeans and soybean products such as tofu.

If your partner avoids dairy products, start buying (or suggest that he start buying) calcium-fortified orange juice. If that doesn't work, consider encouraging him to take a supplement. Calcium carbonate, found in Tums, is an inexpensive and commonly used calcium supplement (take with meals to aid absorption).

The human body needs vitamin D to absorb calcium. Ten minutes of sunshine a day will cause your body to make all the vitamin D it needs. If your partner doesn't get outside much, he can get vitamin D from milk and some fortified breakfast cereals. Otherwise, a multivitamin/mineral supplement will give him the 400 IUs of vitamin D that he needs daily.

Highlighting Homocysteine

A new risk factor for heart disease is emerging. Several studies have found that men and women with higher than average levels of homocysteine, a chemical produced when the body breaks down protein, are at increased risk of heart attack and stroke.

In one study of 15,000 men over a 13-year period, those with the highest levels of homocysteine were three times more likely to have heart attacks than those with the lowest levels.

What role does homocysteine play in the evolution of heart disease? Some researchers believe that high blood levels of this amino acid may injure arterial walls, creating niches in which plaque begins to collect.

Diets high in B vitamins, which are critical to the enzymes that break down homocysteine, have been linked to lower blood levels of the amino acid. It seems logical, then, that eating foods rich in B vitamins will help to protect your heart, although this theory has yet to be tested in a large clinical trial. Good sources of B vitamins include meat, fish, milk products, whole grains, dark green leafy vegetables, and citrus fruits. Most breakfast cereals are fortified with B vitamins.

How Food Affects Cancer Risk

Your body contains billions of cells that carry out all of its functions, which include reproduction, excretion, and metabolism. A control mechanism keeps the number of cells growing in balance with the number of cells dying.

Cancer cells don't respond to this control mechanism. As they reproduce unchecked, they crowd out normal cells and can spread to other parts of the body.

According to the National Cancer Institute, poor diet and obesity cause nearly one-third of all cancer cases. That makes unhealthy eating habits as dangerous as smoking. How does what you eat influence your risk of cancer? Any given food breaks down into many elements, including fat, fiber, phytochemicals, vitamins, minerals, carbohydrates, and protein. Of course, not all of these components play a role in cancer. But many do. Some help prevent the disease from developing; some squelch the growth of existing tumors—and some promote the dreaded disease.

The most studied cancer promoter is fat. Scientists believe that fat may encourage cancer in several ways. Here are three: fatty tissues store cancer-causing chemicals; fat prompts the body to secrete hormones that promote cancer; and fat makes cell membranes vulnerable to cancer-causing agents.

But fat isn't the only culprit. The normal process of metabolism produces harmful molecules called free radicals that can damage tissue. That damage increases cancer risk. Antioxidants, found in fruits and vegetables, neutralize free radicals by mopping them up before they have a chance to do their dirty work. Vitamins C, E, and beta carotene are powerful antioxidants.

When food is processed, other components may be added to preserve them, and to enhance their flavor, texture, and color. These additives are usually present in very small quantities that haven't been linked to human cancers.

However, there's one exception. Some evidence suggests that foods preserved using salt, smoke, and nitrites increase cancer risk. These preservation methods, commonly used for hot dogs, hams, and luncheon meats, can start the cancer ball rolling by introducing carcinogenic (cancer-causing) chemicals into the body.

Once a carcinogen affects a cell, cancerous growth can be encouraged or discouraged by conditions in the body. For example, some researchers believe that linoleic acid, a fat found in vegetable oils, can promote tumor growth. Genistein, a plant chemical found in soybeans and soybean products such as tofu, blocks the formation of blood vessels around new tumors, which cramps their growth.

Diet and Diabetes

Many of us don't worry too much about noninsulin-dependent diabetes—also called Type II or adult-onset diabetes—but we probably should. It can cause such serious complications as heart disease, kidney failure, blindness, and damage to the nervous system. In fact, it's the fourth leading cause of death in the U.S., yet the risk of developing diabetes can be significantly reduced by healthy eating. That means eating plenty of fiber-rich foods and keeping sugary foods to a minimum.

Sugar and highly processed foods increase blood sugar levels, which prompts the pancreas (a gland located behind your stomach) to produce insulin (a hormone that regulates the amount of sugar in the blood). Fiber, on the other hand, decreases the need for insulin. Over time, a high-sugar, low-fiber diet creates a chronic demand for insulin. This strain on the pancreas may lead to diabetes.

Being overweight also can lead to noninsulin dependent diabetes. In fact, between 80 and 90 percent of adults who develop noninsulin dependent diabetes are obese (more than 20 percent above a weight that would be healthy for their height and body type).

WHERE TO FIND OUT MORE

ASSOCIATIONS

• **American Cancer Society.** Address: 1599 Clifton Road, NE, Atlanta, GA 30329. Phone: 1–800–ACS–2345. Internet: http://www.cancer.org. The ACS provides cancer news, research, and information. Its Web site includes links to local chapters.

• **American Diabetes Association.**
Address: 1660 Duke Street, Alexandria, VA 22314. Phone: 1–800–342–2383. Internet: http://www.diabetes.org. The ADA provides diabetes news, information, and resources as well as recipes for people with diabetes. The Web site includes a self-test to help determine an individual's risk for diabetes.

• **American Dietetic Association.**
Address: 216 West Jackson Blvd., Chicago, IL 60606. Phone: 1–312–899–0040. Internet: http://www.eatright.org. This group of registered dietitians provides referrals and information on nutrition research and resources. The Web site includes a daily nutrition tip.

• **American Heart Association.**
Address: 7272 Greenville Avenue, Dallas, TX 75231. Phone: 1–800–242–8721. Internet: http://www.amhrt.org. The AHA offers referrals to cardiologists and support groups as well as journal articles on heart disease and stroke, nutrition information, and heart-healthy recipes.

• **National Heart, Lung, and Blood Institute.**
Address: P.O. Box 30105, Bethesda, MD 20824. Phone: 1–800–575–9355. Internet: http://www.nhlbi.nih.gov/nhlbi/nhlbi.htm. The government's heart institute provides information on a range of cardiovascular topics, recipes, and enrollment information on clinical trials.

WEB SITES

• **DASH (Dietary Approaches to Stop Hypertension) Diet.** Internet: www.dash.bwh.harvard.edu. The site revolves around the DASH diet study and related research. It includes sample menus and tips for following the DASH diet.

• **5 A Day For Better Health.** Internet: www.dcpc.nci.nih.gov/5day/. This site, created as part of a campaign to encourage Americans to eat more fruits and vegetables, is sponsored by the National Cancer Institute and the Produce for Better Health Foundation, a coalition of produce-industry leaders. It features news, research, tips for working five servings of fruits and vegetables into your day, and recipes.

• **Heart Information Network.** Internet: www.heartinfo.com. Features a medical advisory board that can answer questions. Provides articles on heart disease, information on commonly prescribed drugs, and a list of further resources.

Food and Fertility

If fear of having a heart attack isn't enough to get your man to reduce his intake of fat and cholesterol, perhaps this medical tidbit will do the trick: in a study of 3,250 men at the Cooper Clinic in Dallas, those with a total cholesterol of more than 240 mg/dL were 83 percent more likely to have trouble achieving or maintaining an erection than men whose total cholesterol was less than 180 mg/dL.

Just as cholesterol clogs the coronary arteries, it can clog those in the penis. When blood flow becomes impeded, an erection becomes difficult or impossible.

Because body fat plays a role in hormone levels, it can affect fertility. For example, obese men have low testosterone levels and high estrogen levels, a combination that may impede sperm production.

A lack of certain vitamins and minerals is associated with

decreased fertility. For example, too little selenium—a mineral found in brazil nuts, tuna, egg yolks, wheat germ, and some vegetables—can cause infertility.

Too little of the mineral zinc may lead to decreased testosterone production and a low sperm count. Not many meat-eating men are infertile due to a zinc deficiency, but vegetarians may come up short. Oysters are the best source of zinc. Other seafoods, wheat germ, and whole grains also are good sources.

If your partner doesn't get enough vitamin C, his sperm will clump together, a condition called agglutination. Vitamin C is plentiful in citrus fruits, fruit juices, sweet peppers, and strawberries. Vitamin E helps boost libido by keeping testosterone from breaking down. E is present in nuts, seeds, whole grains, fruits, and vegetables. Vegetarians need to make sure they get enough B vitamins, which boost energy and play a role in testosterone production.

What a man eats also affects his sex drive, without which, of course, the issue of fertility would be moot. A healthy diet will help your partner maintain a healthy weight, which usually increases self-confidence and interest in sex. In addition, a healthy diet will give your partner more energy and stamina for sex.

How's that for a good reason to help your man eat healthy?

 TEN TIPS FOR A HEALTHIER DIET
1. Have a piece of fruit and a glass of juice with breakfast every morning.
2. Have fruit for dessert.
3. Make vegetables part of every lunch and dinner.
4. Once a day, snack on a vegetable (try cherry tomatoes, celery, pepper rings, or carrot sticks).

5. Eat red meat no more than three times a week (and remember that 3 ounces of meat is considered a serving).
6. Use skim or 1-percent milk instead of whole or 2-percent.
7. Try eating fat-free yogurt instead of meat at lunch, and use it as a snack.
8. Eat whole grain breads, cereals, pastas, and rice instead of the processed white variety.
9. Use canola or olive oil for cooking and baking.
10. Try a (low-fat) veggieburger at least once.

4

CREATE A HEALTHY KITCHEN

> *It does not matter how slowly you go, as long as you do not stop.*
>
> *Confucius*

So you know the elements of a healthy diet and are, slowly but surely, sharing nutrition information with your man. What next? How do you turn yourself (never mind your partner) into the galloping gourmet of good nutrition? That's the question we'll answer in this chapter. And don't worry, we use the term gourmet loosely. You won't need a subscription to *Martha Stewart Living* or a degree in home economics to pull this off.

That's not to say that changing the way you and your partner eat won't take some thought and planning. But there are many shortcuts to healthy eating, and that's what we'll emphasize here.

Creating a healthy kitchen is a vital part of helping your man get healthier. Why? Because although you can't control what your partner eats, you probably have some measure of control over what his options are—at least at home.

Ava Meade's husband, Bob, who has had two heart attacks, doesn't like it when well-meaning friends or family members comment on what he's eating. "I try not to say anything about what he eats because it bothers him so," says Ava. "Instead, as much as I can, I try to control his diet by what foods I have in the house and how I cook."

To get the ball rolling, invest in a new cookbook or subscribe to a magazine that features healthy recipes. Pick something that will fill a gap in your cooking repertoire. Perhaps you need more information on low-fat cooking (try *Cooking Light* magazine), or maybe you're looking for more ways to use grains, legumes, and vegetables (try *Vegetarian Times*). Soon you'll pick up enough ideas to create healthier versions of your family's favorite meals.

"It takes a lot of time and effort to learn a whole new way of shopping and cooking," says Mary Regan, whose husband, John, had quadruple coronary artery bypass surgery in 1994. "I couldn't just put on a meal anymore. I had to change my whole concept of cooking. I started to read a lot about low-fat eating and went to the nutrition classes offered as part of John's rehabilitation program."

Did her efforts pay off? Five years ago, John was tired more often than not. His diet leaned heavily toward rich desserts and other fatty foods, like beef, liver, bacon, and eggs. He had high blood pressure, for which he was taking medication, and a high serum cholesterol level, for which he was not. At 6 feet 1 inch, he weighed 230 pounds.

One weekend, he was particularly fatigued and complained of a discomfort in his chest that felt like indigestion. When he was evaluated at the local hospital, doctors found that he had 95 percent blockages in four arteries leading to the heart. They scheduled bypass surgery immediately. Shortly after his discharge from the hospital, John and Mary started down the pathway to becoming healthy eaters.

Today, John weighs 200 pounds. His total cholesterol level is 185. His blood pressure is 130/80. "I sleep well and I have loads of energy. You have to want to adopt healthier habits yourself, but I wouldn't be where I am today without Mary. From day one after my surgery, she has cooked only what's good for me." An additional benefit for the Regans is that their three grown children were so inspired by John and Mary's efforts that they've adopted healthier eating habits, too.

HOW TO HANDLE RESISTANCE

What if your partner politely refuses when you offer to slice a banana on top of his bran flakes or gets up to grab some cookies when he sees you coming with a fruit salad? Remind yourself that it's hard for people to change their habits. Take the opportunity to engage your mate in a discussion of which fruits and vegetables are his favorites, which he dislikes, and which he has never tried. Give him his favorites at first, until he's used to the idea of having fruit with breakfast and snacking on vegetables in front of the television. Once that becomes a habit for both of you, try experimenting with a wider variety of fruits and vegetables. Remember, gradual change, in this case through gradual food substitution, leads to permanent changes.

If your partner hasn't been receptive to the idea that you should both try to eat more produce, don't push the issue. If you do that, he's more likely to dig in and refuse all the harder. Instead, your best course of action is to lead by example. As Henry David Thoreau once said: "If you would convince a man that he does wrong, do right. Men will believe what they see." The fact that you have changed your eating habits will eventually make an impression on him. He'll be inspired by your understanding of how to become a healthy eater and by your dedication, some of which is bound to rub off on him.

Go at Your Own Pace

As you and your partner set about changing your diets, the first question you'll need to answer is whether you'll find it easier to change gradually or all at once. This will depend on each partner's personality and medical circumstances. Some people prefer to alter their eating habits radically rather than to extend the change process over several months or a year. They find the former exciting and challenging; the latter dull. Others need to make significant changes quickly because they're facing an immediate health threat.

After her husband, Danny, had his second heart attack at age 37, Marcia Shainis of Wilton, Connecticut, changed her cooking habits almost overnight. "I threw out everything that wasn't part of a low-fat diet," she says. "I turned the whole kitchen upside down and learned a whole new way of food shopping and cooking."

People who aren't faced with an immediate health threat may feel more comfortable making changes at a slower pace. Pat Corbett of Brewster, Massachusetts, took the gradual approach to change. "In the beginning, I just made a few healthy changes for myself," she explains. "For example, I stopped drinking soda and started drinking water. My two daughters and my husband followed suit in their own time. What my family sees me do, they want to do. They think that if I'm doing it for myself, it must be good."

Over time, the family diet has become healthier in many ways. These days, dinner at the Corbetts always includes fruits and vegetables and usually features chicken or a vegetarian dish rather than red meat. The Corbetts routinely snack on fresh fruit and sliced raw vegetables instead of cookies, and they drink skim instead of whole milk.

"Cooking was all trial and tribulation in the beginning," says Pat. "Things didn't always come out right. I just did what I could until things came easier. Then I was able to experiment a little to find meals that worked well for us."

Every family needs to find dishes that suit its lifestyle and taste buds. Trial and error is really the only way to come up with these meals. Keep experimenting until you have a variety of options for snacks, breakfasts, lunches, and dinners. Mary Regan learned a lesson from her mother that she has applied to the process of changing her husband's diet. "My mom told me two things about cooking for children: you have to make the food palatable and you have to have variety. I've found that the same rules apply to preparing food for John. Everyone wants to enjoy the food they eat and everyone needs variety."

John agrees: "Mary makes it taste good," he says. "I have so much chicken, but I never have the same chicken twice."

 TEN QUICK HEALTHY MEALS

If you and your partner are like many couples, you don't have time to spend an hour cooking dinner every night. But that doesn't mean your meals can't be healthy. Here are 10 examples of dinners (or lunches) that are almost preparation-free but still good for you.

1. Canned, low-salt, bean or vegetable soup served with fresh, whole-grain bread and a salad.

2. Canned, low-salt, vegetarian chili served over a baked potato. Steam your favorite frozen vegetables and stir them into the chili or serve them on the side. If you don't want to use canned chili, add low-fat, ground turkey breast or a soy meat substitute to a can of tomato sauce, a can of kidney beans (rinsed), and an envelope of chili seasoning.

3. Black bean burritos made as follows: Mix 1 can of black beans (rinsed to remove excess salt) with ½ cup salsa. Spoon filling into the center of whole-wheat tortillas, then roll up the tortillas (secure with toothpicks if necessary). Place on a baking sheet. Sprinkle with low-fat or fat-free cheese. Bake in the oven for 20 minutes at 350 degrees. If you don't like tortillas, serve the bean and salsa mixture over rice.

4. Sauté sliced fresh or frozen vegetables with garlic in a little olive oil and soy sauce. Serve over pasta or brown rice. If you like, serve meat on the side (about 3 ounces per person). Choose a lean cut such as eye of round, top round, or round tip.

5. Place boneless, skinless, chicken breast (about ¼ pound per person) in a baking pan that has been coated with a nonstick spray. Bake for 20 minutes at 350 degrees. Top each piece with one of the following: white-wine Worcestershire sauce, sweet and sour sauce, pizza sauce, barbecue sauce, or honey mustard (look for low-sodium brands). Cook another 10 minutes or until chicken is done and sauce is hot. Serve with a salad or steamed fresh or frozen vegetables.

6. Place sole fillets (¼ pound per person) in a baking pan. Add ¼ cup white wine or chicken broth. Top fillets with a little Molly McButter, pepper, dried parsley, and lemon slices (at least one slice per fillet). Bake at 450 degrees for 10 minutes or until fish flakes easily. Serve with a salad or steamed vegetables.

7. Make your own pizza. Use frozen pizza dough, low salt pizza sauce and low fat or fat free cheese. Top with sliced vegetables (try carrots, broccoli, mushrooms, garlic, peppers, tomatoes). Bake per directions on dough package.

8. Combine canned beans or lentils (rinsed) with cooked vegetables and pasta. Top with your favorite low-sodium pasta sauce. In the summer, use raw vegetables and serve chilled with your favorite low-fat dressing.

9. Try veggieburgers. You'll probably find several varieties in your grocery store. Some taste better than others, so don't give up after sampling just one. You might share with a neighbor, each buying a different brand, so that you can try several without ending up with a freezer full of half-empty boxes of veggieburgers. Check the nutrition label, because some brands are surprisingly high in fat.

10. Baste salmon or tuna steaks with 2 parts lemon juice to 1 part olive oil. Grill under the broiler or over charcoal. Serve with boiled red potatoes and your favorite vegetables (steamed).

To Market, to Market

Healthy eating starts with healthy food shopping, so we'll begin our lesson on creating a healthy kitchen with a trip to the grocery store. As Marcia Shainis points out: "You can learn a lot from going through a grocery store and just looking at nutrition labels." So we'll start with a look at labels.

The Nutrition Facts listed on packaged foods tell you what you need to know to make smart food choices. Look for products that are low in fat (especially saturated fat), cholesterol, sodium, and sugar. Choose items that are high in fiber and complex carbohydrates. (To determine whether a food is high in complex carbohydrates, subtract the number of grams of sugar from the number of grams listed next to "total carbohydrate.")

Because high fat intake has been linked to heart disease, cancer, and stroke, experts recommend that we get no more than 30 percent of daily calories from fat. That means choosing individual foods that, on average, derive no more than 30 percent of calories from fat.

Use the food label to determine what proportion of your daily fat allowance a given product will contribute. Simply divide the number of calories per serving by 30. For example, a serving of whole milk contains 150 calories. Dividing 150 by 30 gives you 5. Thus, to fall within the recommended range, a serving of milk should have no more than 5 grams of fat. Whole milk has 8 grams.

SAMPLE NUTRITION LABEL

Serving size reflects the amounts people usually eat. (If you eat more than the serving size listed, adjust the % daily values accordingly.)

The list of nutrients covers those most important to the health of today's consumers.

Nutrition Facts

Serving Size ½ cup (114g)
Servings Per Container 4

Amount Per Serving

Calories 90	Calories from Fat 30

% Daily Value*

Total Fat 3g	**5%**
Saturated Fat 0g	**0%**
Cholesterol 0mg	**0%**
Sodium 300mg	**13%**
Total Carbohydrate 13g	**4%**
Dietary Fiber 3g	**12%**
Sugars 3g	
Protein 3g	

Vitamin A	80%	•	Vitamin C	60%
Calcium	4%	•	Iron	4%

* Percent Daily Values are based on a 2,000 calorie diet. Your daily values may be higher or lower depending on your calorie needs:

	Calories	2,000	2,500
Total Fat	Less than	65g	80g
Sat Fat	Less than	20g	25g
Cholesterol	Less than	300mg	300mg
Sodium	Less than	2,400mg	2,400mg
Total Carbohydrate		300g	375g
Fiber		25g	30g

Calories per gram:
Fat 9   •   Carbohydrate 4   •   Protein 4

Calories from Fat are shown on the label to help consumers meet dietary guidelines that recommend people get no more than 30 percent of the calories in their overall diet from fat.

% Daily Value (DV) shows how a food in the specified serving size fits into the overall daily diet. By using **% DV** you can easily determine whether a food contributes a lot or little of a particular nutrient. And you can compare different foods with no need to do any calculations.

Source: Report of the Dietary Guidelines Advisory Committee on the Dietary Guidelines for Americans, 1995, to the Secretary of Health and Human Services and the Secretary of Agriculture

When reading food labels, be aware that there are several types of dietary fat and that some are harder on your health than others. (See: "Fat: The Good, the Bad, and the Ugly" on page 132.) One type of fat we haven't yet mentioned is hydrogenated fat. Hydrogenated fat is a polyunsaturated fat that contains trans-fatty acids. Trans-fatty acids should be avoided because they act like saturated fat, increasing LDLs and decreasing HDLs. Hydrogenated fat is created when food manufacturers turn liquid fat into a solid form such as stick margarine.

Here's a simple rule of thumb: fat that's liquid at room temperature (vegetable oil) is better for your health than fat that's solid at room temperature (stick margarine, Crisco, animal fat). Why? Because solid fats are more likely to contain saturated or hydrogenated fat.

Produce Planning

In most stores, the first aisle you come to is the produce aisle. This area is, of course, chock full of foods that can supply the vitamins, minerals, and other nutrients your body needs for good health.

Because fresh vegetables and fruits don't stay fresh for extended periods of time, it's best to plan ahead. Shop from a list that you made at home after considering the following variables: what you want for dinner for the next several nights; what you already have on hand; and who will be around to eat it. (If you or your partner will be away on business or having dinner with a friend one night, take that into account). The list will help to prevent impulse buying of additional fruits and vegetables than may languish in the refrigerator, eventually going bad.

Plan for three or four days' worth of fruits and vegetables, then restock midweek. This may mean an extra trip to the grocery store, but if you go in with a list and need to visit only the produce department, it'll be a quick trip. This midweek restocking will ensure that the foods that are "good for you" will always be fresh, bright, crisp, and attractive to look at as well as to taste.

What should you choose from the produce aisle? First and foremost, choose what you and your family like. Trying to convert a broccoli hater into a broccoli lover will probably discourage you and increase your partner's negative feelings about vegetables.

Experiment with new or more exotic fruits and vegetables periodically. How often you do so will depend on how adventurous you and your partner are. For most people, the top priority should be eating *more* fruits and vegetables. Once that becomes a habit, your goal can be to eat a wider variety.

 FOODS THAT FIGHT BACK
According to the U.S. Department of Agriculture, the following fruits and vegetables have the greatest antioxidant activity in laboratory tests:

1. Blueberries
2. Kale
3. Strawberries
4. Spinach
5. Brussels sprouts
6. Plums
7. Broccoli
8. Beets
9. Oranges
10. Red grapes

Best Bets in the Produce Aisle

Although you'd be hard pressed to make an unhealthy choice in the produce aisle, some vegetables and fruits are more nutritious than others. The most obvious example lies in the green, leafy vegetables. Generally, the darker the leaves, the more nutrients contained therein. For example, iceberg lettuce, with its almost-white leaves, is the least nutritious of the greens. In fact, it's mainly water, which may be why it's called "iceberg" lettuce. Romaine lettuce has a texture similar to that of iceberg but is more nutritious.

The nutritional star of this group is arugula, a lettuce family member that has small flat leaves resembling those of the dandelion. Arugula contains the most beta carotene (4 mg per 3.5 ounces), the most vitamin C (91 mg) and the most calcium (309 mg) of any of the green leafy vegetables. It has a peppery taste and is most often used as a salad green, but it also can be used in pasta sauce, soup, or poultry stuffing.

Among both sweet and hot peppers, red peppers contain more vitamin C and beta carotene than do green peppers. Among red peppers, hot varieties contain almost twice as much vitamin A, beta carotene, and vitamin C as do sweet varieties. When it comes to winter squashes (acorn, butternut, hubbard, pumpkin, and spaghetti), butternut has the most beta carotene and vitamin C.

You'll find differences among similar fruits, too. The varieties of avocado that are grown in California have almost twice the fat (about 17g) of those grown in Florida (about 9g). Red grapefruit has enough beta carotene to supply 12 percent of the recommended daily allowance for vitamin A; white grapefruit has only a trace of beta carotene. Among melons, cantaloupe packs the most nutrients.

GIVE YOUR MAN GARLIC?

These days, it seems garlic is on everyone's breath. What's all the excitement about, and is it warranted? This vegetable seems to provide three types of protection against heart disease: it lowers blood pressure, lowers total cholesterol, and helps to prevent blood clots by making platelets (a cell-like element in the blood that's essential for clotting) less sticky. That's important because too much of a good thing, like clotting when you get a cut, is bad.

The downside? Studies indicate that you would have to eat a relatively large amount of garlic to reap its rewards. To top things off, some experts believe that cooking decreases the amount of the compound thought to be responsible for garlic's health benefits. If that turns out to be true, eating several cloves of raw garlic daily would be the only way to take advantage of its promise.

Garlic supplements come in pill, powder and capsule form, but they aren't necessarily a solution. Because the supplements aren't regulated, they vary widely in strength and quality. Scientists don't yet know whether the supplements provide the same benefits as the real thing. The heat applied in the manufacturing process may destroy garlic's active compounds.

Until more studies are done, your best bet may be to cook with garlic frequently—if you and your partner *both* enjoy it. If one partner abstains from garlic, the other would be well advised not to indulge too heartily. Garlic's pungent odor may send even the most loving partner to the far side of the bed. If garlic doesn't have a future in your kitchen, try using more onions when you cook—they appear to offer some of the same health benefits.

Coming to Terms with Convenience

Fresh fruits and vegetables begin to loose nutrient value once cut, so it's better (and cheaper) to buy them whole. However, don't hesitate to take advantage of conveniences like packaged salads and presliced vegetables if that's the only way they'll make it onto your lunch, dinner, or snack plate. Once you and your partner get into the habit of eating more vegetables, you may be more inclined to take on the task of washing and cutting them up yourselves.

If convenience is important for you, use frozen or canned vegetables and fruits. You can keep them on hand for extended periods (thus cutting down on midweek trips to the supermarket), and they come ready to cook or eat. Although taste and texture may not be at the level of fresh produce, in most cases the nutritional quality doesn't suffer. In fact, some canned or frozen fruits and vegetables provide more vitamins than their fresh counterparts.

For example, frozen or canned asparagus contains significantly more vitamin A and C than does asparagus bought fresh at the supermarket. Canned pumpkin has much more vitamin A than does fresh cooked pumpkin. One possible explanation is that frozen and canned vegetables are processed within hours of harvest, locking in vital nutrients. "Fresh" produce, on the other hand, may have been harvested as many as 25 days before you buy it in the supermarket. A couple of caveats: when buying canned fruit, pick brands packed in fruit juice instead of syrup. The latter contains extra sugar. When buying canned vegetables, look for brands that are low in sodium.

Go Nuts!

In the produce aisle, you may find nuts, seeds, and dried fruits available in bulk bins from which you serve yourself into plastic bags (look for prepackaged nuts and seeds in the snack aisle and for prepackaged dried fruits in the baking aisle). Most of these items are healthy. Although nuts and seeds are high in fat, the fat is mostly unsaturated, so it won't raise blood cholesterol. Do avoid coconuts, Brazil nuts, macadamias, and cashews, which are especially high in saturated fat.

Peanuts, which are actually legumes (edible seeds enclosed in a pod), are a good source of protein on their own. Other nuts are good sources of protein when consumed together with legumes or animal products. Nuts are high in vitamins and minerals, including vitamin E, B vitamins (thiamin, niacin, and riboflavin), potassium, iron, magnesium, zinc, copper, and selenium. Seeds are good sources of iron, potassium, phosphorus, and fiber, especially when eaten with their hulls.

Fruits that are commonly offered in dried form include grapes (raisins), plums (prunes), apples, apricots, bananas, dates, figs, peaches, and pineapples. Dried fruits are high in sugar and calories, but they're also high in iron, copper, potassium, beta carotene, and fiber.

Nuts, seeds, and dried fruits are good snacks for people who are on the go and might otherwise grab a few cookies (most of which are high in fat) on their way out the door. Your partner can keep a mix of his favorites in his briefcase or desk drawer at work to ward off trips to the vending machine. Dried fruits can be added to hot or cold breakfast cereal; nuts and seeds can be used to add vitamins and minerals to stir-fry dishes and whole-grain breads and muffins.

Shopping for a Multivitamin

The next aisle we'll visit is health and beauty aids, home of vitamin and mineral supplements. The big question here is, of course, whether healthy adults need a supplement. Although women of childbearing age have to be sure they get enough of several special nutrients (such as folic acid, calcium, and iron), men aren't under the same pressure.

THIRTY WAYS TO EAT MORE FRUIT AND VEGETABLES

Although most of us know that fruits and vegetables are good for us, we don't eat the recommended amount (at least five servings daily). To help you increase your consumption, we've compiled a list of simple ways you and your partner (and any children you may have) can make produce an integral part of your daily diet.

BREAKFAST

1. Drink juice every morning. Six ounces of 100-percent fruit juice equals one serving. That amount of orange or grapefruit juice more than fulfills your body's daily demand for vitamin C.

2. Top hot or cold cereal with fruit. Try blueberries, raisins, sliced bananas or strawberries, and diced apples. Canned fruits work, too—try peaches and mandarins.

3. Add fruit to pancake batter or serve pancakes topped with fruit. (Try blueberries, sliced bananas or strawberries, and mandarin orange sections.)

4. Top low-fat vanilla yogurt with fresh or frozen (thawed) berries.

5. Eat one-third of a cantaloupe melon, half a grapefruit, or a bowl of pineapple chunks with your breakfast.

6. Make an omelet with one or more vegetables. (Try onions, tomatoes, peppers, mushrooms, broccoli, and asparagus.)

7. Mix arugula into low-fat cream cheese and spread it on a whole-grain bagel.

LUNCH

8. Top your sandwich with tomatoes, cucumber, dark-green lettuce leaves, or onions.

9. Eat vegetable soup (add potatoes or pasta for a heartier meal).

10. Eat a salad with raw vegetables added. Try red or green peppers, sliced or shredded carrots, broccoli, cucumber, tomato, or whatever is left from last night's dinner.

11. Add vegetables to pasta salad. Try the same ideas as for a green salad.

12. To add texture to a salad, use kidney beans or chickpeas instead of croutons.

13. Make a bean or vegetable salad. Try three-bean salad (fresh green beans, kidney beans, and chickpeas are a good combination) or tomato and green bean salad. Top with your favorite store-bought or homemade low-fat dressing.

14. Make a fruit and vegetable salad. Try adding raisins, chopped apples, grapefruit, or orange sections to arugula or romaine lettuce. Mix shredded carrot with raisins and top with a vinaigrette dressing.

15. Top a baked potato with low-fat cheese and a vegetable of your choice. This is a great way to make use of leftover vegetables.

16. Make a side dish of your favorite vegetable.
17. Eat fresh fruit for dessert. If you're helping your partner pack his lunch for work, choose easy-to-eat fruits such as apples, pears, and peaches. (Don't forget to include a napkin.)

Dinner

18. Serve raw vegetables (with salsa or a low-fat dip), vegetable soup, or a cold fruit soup (in summer) as an appetizer.
19. Add vegetables to pasta sauce. A half-cup of tomato sauce counts as one serving of vegetables. Adding a half-cup of sliced vegetables will bring you up to two servings. Try asparagus, onion, broccoli, peas, green beans, or a mixture of your favorites. If your partner is leery of vegetables, grate or chop them finely before adding to the sauce (carrots and zucchini work well).
20. Add extra vegetables to casseroles, stews, and lasagna.
21. Serve a side dish of vegetables *and* a salad.
22. Cut lean beef, chicken, or fish into pieces and put it on a skewer, alternating it with vegetables such as onions, cherry tomatoes, mushrooms, and sweet peppers. Broil or grill the kebabs for three to five minutes per side (about 4 inches from the heat).
23. Eat fruit for dessert. Fruit looks more like a dessert and will be more readily eaten by those at the table if it has been sliced or cut up into bite-sized pieces beforehand. So slice and core apples and pears, make melon balls, peel and cut up oranges and kiwi.

Snacks

24. Top plain or vanilla yogurt with fresh fruit.
25. Cut up raw vegetables and store them in a plastic bag in plain view in the refrigerator. Cherry tomatoes make a great snack, too.
26. Keep a bowl on the counter stocked with your family's favorite fruits.
27. Cut some fruit up and leave it on the coffee table before the movie or big game.
28. Add extra vegetables to store-bought chunky-style salsa. Try chopped cucumber or zucchini. Use fat-free crackers or baked tortilla chips for dipping.
29. Keep a bag of dried fruit in your car or in your desk drawer at work. Suggest that your partner do the same.
30. Mix unsalted nuts or pretzels with raisins or dried apricots.

Why? For a start, they don't bear children or menstruate, activities that increase a woman's nutritional needs. Another reason is simply that men eat more than women, so they have more chances to get the nutrients they need from food.

Food is the best place to get the nutrients your body needs, but you and your partner may want to use supplements while you're revamping your diet. Once you reach five or more servings of fruits and vegetables per day and are eating lots of legumes, whole grains, and low-fat dairy products, you can give them up. In the meantime, a little insurance won't hurt. Also, continuing to use a supplement in a modest dosage won't hurt either.

Don't share a supplement. Men and women have different nutritional needs. For example, most men get plenty of iron in their diets, so they should select a supplement without added iron (too much iron can be harmful). Women, on the other hand, may want a little extra iron because they typically consume less than men and they loose some each month during menstruation. One possible exception is if your partner is a vegetarian—he may not be getting enough iron. Still, choose a supplement with no more than 10 milligrams of iron.

Don't go for a supplement that promises 10 times the Recommended Daily Allowance (RDA) for everything. More isn't necessarily better. In fact, large doses of some nutrients, including zinc, selenium, manganese, phosphorus, iron, niacin, and vitamins A, B_6, and D, can be harmful. Stick to a multivitamin that gives you no more than 100 percent of the RDA (also called the daily value or DV) for most vitamins and minerals. (See "Supplements: Don't Take Too Much of a Good Thing" on page 128.)

Having trouble convincing your man to take a multivitamin? You may be using the wrong approach. A market-research firm in Florida found that men and women take vitamins for different reasons. Women take vitamins because they believe that doing so will boost their energy level and improve their appearance (an unlikely outcome, actually). Men are more interested in improving their fitness level and reducing the negative effects of stress. While there is little evidence that any vitamin or mineral has a direct effect on fitness levels or the ability to handle stress, supplements can help indirectly by providing the body with the RDA for the nutrients it needs to stay healthy. Try telling your partner that a multivitamin can help ensure that his body has the resources it needs to handle everyday physical and mental challenges.

SUPPLEMENTS:
DON'T TAKE TOO MUCH OF A GOOD THING

Vitamins and minerals are good for us, right? Sure, but as with so much in life, moderation is key. The Council for Responsible Nutrition, an association of the dietary supplement industry, has published scientifically reviewed guidelines that list safe levels of various nutrients. It's important to note that these levels include intake from both food and supplements. Use the table below to steer clear of multivitamins that pack too big a punch.

Nutrient	Safe Level for Daily Consumption
Vitamin A	10,000 IU (International Units)
Vitamin B_6	200 mg (milligrams)
Vitamin B_{12}	3,000 mcg (micrograms)
Folic acid	1,000 mcg
Vitamin C	1,000 mg
Vitamin D	800 IU

Nutrient	Safe Level for Daily Consumption
Vitamin E	800 mg
Calcium	1,500 mg
Chromium	1,000 mcg
Iron	65 mg
Magnesium	700 mg
Selenium	200 mcg
Zinc	30 mg

Choosing Condiments

The condiment aisle in the supermarket offers several opportunities to reduce the fat in your family's diet. Most of the reduced-fat options will leave you feeling deprived only temporarily, if at all. It doesn't take long to get used to low-fat mayonnaise, for example. Or start using mustard instead of mayonnaise on sandwiches. Another alternative: Hellmann's Dijonnaise, described as a fat-free "creamy mustard blend." As the name suggests, it tastes like a cross between mustard and mayonnaise.

Buy a reduced-fat variety of your partner's favorite salad dressing. If he likes that, you might eventually try a fat-free dressing. Or, as a compromise, buy one fat free and one reduced fat bottle, mix them, and serve. Stock up on salsa. It's a good source of lycopene, an antioxidant found in tomatoes that reduces prostate-cancer risk.

Don't Bypass the Beans

Making beans a regular part of your diet can reduce risk of colorectal cancers, heart disease, and diabetes. Dried beans and other legumes, such as split peas and lentils, are low in fat and are excellent sources of fiber, carbohydrates, and protein. Canned beans can be high in fat, so check labels.

With the exception of soybeans and peanuts, legumes

don't provide a complete protein, but that problem is easily remedied by serving legumes with rice or a small amount of an animal product (poultry, fish, eggs, or low-fat yogurt). Legumes are also good sources of B vitamins, zinc, potassium, magnesium, calcium, and iron.

In addition to offering a complete protein, soybeans provide fiber and other essential nutrients, including calcium, zinc, iron, and several of the B vitamins. Although soybeans are higher in fat than other legumes, the fat is mostly "healthy" unsaturated fat.

There's much epidemiologic evidence suggesting that people who eat a lot of soy products have very low rates of several cancers, especially those of the breast, prostate, colon, and endometrium (lining of the uterus). Soy also has been shown to reduce LDL ("bad") cholesterol and triglycerides without reducing HDL ("good") cholesterol. Some researchers believe that soy protein can protect women from osteoporosis and help to prevent menopausal symptoms such as hot flashes.

Typically, soybeans aren't used in their natural form. Most often, they're processed into soy milk, tofu (a soft cheeselike food that can be used as a meat or cheese substitute in stir-fries, casseroles, soups, puddings, and cheesecakes), and various other meat substitutes. Soybean oil is used in cooking and in making margarine and salad dressings. Other soy products include breakfast cereal, cream substitute (for coffee and gravies), butter (resembles peanut butter), flour, cheese, yogurt, miso (a salty paste that can be used in soups, stews, sauces, dips, and gravies), and tempeh (a dense, chewy cake that can be grilled, fried, or steamed for use as a meat substitute). If you want recipes that use soy foods, borrow or buy a vegetarian cookbook.

Some soy products are probably available at your local

supermarket. Look for a wider selection of products at health food stores and Asian markets. Or order by mail from a health-foods company (such as Dixie U.S.A.; phone: 1–800–347–3494).

Keep a supply of your favorite legumes on hand. Plan ahead if you're using dried legumes—most should be soaked overnight before cooking. Also rinse canned beans to reduce salt content.

Here are some ways to use common legumes. Try black beans in soup or burritos. Use mashed chickpeas to make hummus (a spread for crackers or sandwiches). Add cannellini (large, white kidney beans) to soup or pasta sauce. Use red kidney beans to make chili; split peas to make soup. Legumes, including red kidney beans, lentils, and chickpeas, can enhance a tossed salad by adding texture and nutrients.

Pick a Peck of Pasta

Load up on your favorite types of pasta to use as the basis for hundreds of healthy meals. Pasta is rich in complex carbohydrates, high in protein, low in fat—and easy to prepare. Cook pasta in plenty of water to avoid sticking. Don't add salt when cooking—you won't miss it. Reheat leftover pasta in a microwave or by dropping it into boiling water for 30 seconds. An alternative is to toss leftover pasta with light or fat-free Italian dressing and store it in an airtight container in the refrigerator for a day or two. It can be added to a green salad or tossed with vegetables to make a pasta salad.

Stock up on Rice

Rice is another good source of carbohydrates and other important nutrients. It's high in both soluble and insoluble fiber, B vitamins (such as thiamin and niacin), and iron. Wild rice, brown rice, and parboiled (also called converted) rice are the most nutritious choices because they include the husks, which contain most of rice's nutrients. These forms offer more of several important nutrients, including fiber, folacin, riboflavin, potassium, phosphorus, and trace minerals such as copper and manganese, than enriched white rice, from which the husks have been removed.

If you buy preseasoned rice, check the salt content. Even if you're not on a salt-restricted diet, choose a brand with no more than about 500 milligrams of sodium per serving. If you are on a salt-restricted diet, look for brands with no salt added or avoid preseasoned rices altogether.

Use the same sodium guidelines when choosing a ready-made pasta sauce. Avoid brands that list cream or cheese as ingredients, but don't go nuts looking for a totally fat-free variety. Here's why: tomatoes are rich in lycopene, an antioxidant that appears to reduce the risk of prostate cancer. The lycopene in tomatoes is better absorbed by the body when they're cooked in a little oil. In one study, volunteers who ate tomato sauce cooked in oil got roughly 10 times more lycopene into their systems as did volunteers who drank tomato juice that contained the same amount of lycopene but no oil.

FAT: THE GOOD, THE BAD, AND THE UGLY

Contrary to what many Americans now believe, some fats are actually good for you. Specifically, monounsaturated fat lowers LDL cholesterol levels but leaves beneficial HDL cholesterol intact, and may even increase it. Still, this type of fat should account for just 10 to 13 percent of daily calories.

Polyunsaturated fat is the next least harmful: It reduces both "good" and "bad" cholesterol levels. This type of fat should make up no more than 10 percent of daily calories.

Saturated fat is the one you really want to avoid: It raises the level of harmful LDL cholesterol in your blood. In a healthy diet, no more than 7 to 10 percent of daily calories should come from saturated fats. That means limiting red meat and foods such as butter, whole milk, cheese, ice cream, and oils such as coconut, palm, and cottonseed.

Use the table below to choose healthier fats for yourself and your mate.

Type of Fat	% Saturated	% Polyunsaturated	% Monounsaturated
Canola oil	6	32	62
Safflower oil	10	77	13
Sunflower oil	11	69	20
Corn oil	13	62	25
Olive oil	14	9	77
Soybean oil	15	61	24
Margarine (tub)	17	34	24
Peanut oil	18	33	49
Cottonseed oil	27	54	19
Chicken fat	31	22	47
Lard	41	12	47
Beef fat	52	4	44
Palm kernel oil	81	2	11
Coconut oil	92	2	6

Source: *Compositions of Foods*, U.S. Department of Agriculture

Be Wary When Selecting Snacks

There are some reasonably healthy foods hidden among the fat-laden treats in the snack aisle. Most pretzels are fat-free. Salt-free pretzels are an even better choice. "Lite" popcorn is a fairly healthy snack because it's low in fat and contains a lot of fiber. Again, however, watch the sodium content. Most stores stock a variety of fat-free baked chips, which are certainly worth trying instead of regular potato chips.

A common mistake among dieters today is overindulging in "fat-free" cookies, cakes, and ice creams. It's important to remember that fat-free isn't calorie-free. If your man habitually overdoses on reduced fat treats, he won't loose weight. And he'll be filling up on foods that don't provide the nutrients his body needs.

Breakfast of Champions

Breakfast is the most important meal of the day because it follows a 10- or 12-hour overnight fast. Compared to those who don't bother with breakfast, people who eat in the morning tend to have stronger problem-solving skills and more energy early in the day. They also tend to eat less at lunch and dinner, and to have healthier diets, lower cholesterol and fat levels, and fewer excess pounds. Despite the many benefits of breakfast, about a quarter of Americans skip it altogether.

Let's face it, mornings are frantic for most of us. But there are ways to fit breakfast in with minimal fuss. Cold cereal is fast, healthy, and tastes good (with all those varieties, there's got to be at least one that you and your partner like). Look for a brand that's low in fat (2 grams or less per serving); low in sugar (6 grams or less); high in fiber (at least 2 grams) and high in protein (at least 3 grams). Other reasons to opt for breakfast cereals is that they're fortified with essential vitamins and minerals, and you eat them with milk, which provides much needed calcium and vitamin D.

If your man says he isn't hungry in the morning, help

him get in the breakfast habit by eating a little something each morning for two weeks. He might try a breakfast bar with a glass of milk or a piece of fruit and a slice of toast to get started. Once his body adjusts to this new eating habit, he can aim for a more complete morning meal that consists of, say, a bowl of cereal with milk and a glass of juice.

To help keep your partner in the breakfast habit, make sure the cereal you select not only is healthy but also tastes good. Also, keep more than one variety on hand to prevent breakfast boredom. Suggest that your partner try mixing a high-fiber cereal (more than 5 grams) with his favorite cereal (as long as that's not Captain Crunch).

Selecting Seafood

When you arrive at the seafood counter, consider buying some salmon. It's rich in heart-healthy omega-3 fatty acids. So rich, in fact, that William Castelli, M.D., retired head of the Framingham Heart Study, recommends that his patients eat salmon twice a week. If you don't care for salmon, pick up one of the other fatty fishes—tuna, swordfish, sardines, or mackerel. Leaner varieties of fish are healthy, too, of course. High in protein and B vitamins, fish is always a healthy alternative to red meat.

Looking for an easy way to add fish to your diet? Make a tuna- or salmon-salad sandwich. Mix canned tuna or salmon (packed in water) with a little low-fat mayonnaise. Add some celery, red pepper, or any other chopped vegetable for variety.

WHY FISH FAT IS GOOD FOR YOU

Fatty fish like salmon, swordfish, mackerel, blue fish, tuna, herring, anchovies and sardines contain omega-3 fatty acids. These polyunsaturated fats act as blood-thinners, which means they help to prevent the blood clots that can cause heart attack and stroke. Omega-3s also have been found to lower blood pressure as well as the total amount of fat in the blood as measured by triglycerides. When triglycerides decrease, production of HDL cholesterol increases.

How much fish do you have to eat to reap the rewards? A 30-year study of 1,800 Chicago-area men found that those who ate at least eight ounces (two to three servings) of fish a week had a 40 percent lower risk of fatal heart attack than those who ate no fish.

You may have heard or read about fish oil supplements, but unless your partner's doctor has recommended them, he's better off sticking to food sources of omega-3s. Fish-oil supplements may overly thin the blood, delaying clotting. For that reason, the American Heart Association recommends that supplements be used "only for patients who have high levels of triglycerides in the blood that cannot be lowered by drug treatment and who are at increased risk for pancreatitis."

Choosing Healthier Cuts of Meat and Poultry

At the meat counter, choose "select" grades of round steak, flank steak, sirloin tip, tenderloin, or "extra lean" (also called "90-percent lean") ground beef. If you're shopping for pork, ask for tenderloin, loin chops, rib or loin roasts, or low-fat ham. When it comes to lamb, choose leg sirloin chop, center roast, center slice, or shank. If you're buying veal, ask for leg cutlet, arm steak, sirloin steak, rib chop, loin chop, or top round.

If you're having chicken or turkey, choose white meat over dark—it's significantly lower in fat. Poultry skin is very high in fat, so always remove the skin before eating.

THE LEANEST OF MEATS

You don't have to give up meat to call your diet healthy. Just stick to these low fat choices whenever possible.

Type of Meat	Fat (g)
Skinless turkey breast	1
Skinless chicken breast	4
Veal leg	4
Skinless turkey drumstick	4
Beef eye of round, minute steak	5
Skinless chicken drumstick	6
Beef top round, London broil	6
Pork tenderloin	7
Beef top loin, strip steak	7
Veal shoulder, loin or sirloin	7
Lamb shank	8
Pork chop	8
Beef sirloin	9

Making Smart Dairy Decisions

The dairy case provides ample opportunity to get good nutrition with little or no fat. If you're not already drinking skim milk, make that one of your goals. Start now by buying milk that's one fat level below the milk you currently drink. For example, if you drink 2-percent milk, switch to 1-percent. Once you get used to that, trade down to skim. Making the switch gradually virtually guarantees that you'll be successful.

That's how the Corbett family got used to skim milk. "Now skim milk is all we buy," says Pat. "One day, my husband came home with 1-percent milk because the store was out of skim. Both of our daughters looked up from their cereal at the same time and said: 'There's something wrong with the milk.' "

You can use the same technique for milk products, including cheese, cottage cheese, and yogurt. Start with a low-fat version, then eventually try a fat-free version. Even if you never make it to the fat-free level, using reduced fat products will spare you a lot of damaging saturated fat.

A word about yogurt: if you and your partner aren't in the habit of eating yogurt, try to incorporate it into your diet. Low-fat or nonfat yogurt is an excellent source of calcium and protein, and a good source of riboflavin, phosphorus, and vitamin B_{12}. Add your own fruit to plain, vanilla, or lemon yogurt, and you've got part of a delicious and healthy breakfast, mid-afternoon snack, or after-dinner treat. Be aware that fruit-flavored yogurts are high in sugar. Plain yogurt can be used in many different ways. Some examples are as a substitute for mayonnaise, heavy cream, whipped cream, or sour cream.

Refrigerated fruit juices are usually found near the dairy products. Juice should be a part of every breakfast. There are so many varieties available that one is sure to tickle your man's taste buds. Because most men and women don't get enough calcium, consider choosing an orange juice that's fortified with this important mineral. Each glass of calcium-enriched juice contains as much calcium as a glass of milk.

Easy on the Eggs

Eggs, while not as terrible for our health as we were once led to believe, should be used sparingly because they are high in fat and cholesterol. Try using an egg substitute for pancakes, muffins, and other baked goods. If you like those things (you probably won't notice the difference), try making an omelet or scrambled eggs with the egg substitute.

When you do use eggs, consider using Egg-Land's Best, or a type that's similar. These eggs come from hens who have been fed a vegetarian diet enriched with vitamin E. The result? Eggs that contain more vitamin E (25 percent of the RDA versus 4 percent in ordinary eggs) and a little less cholesterol (195 milligrams on average versus 213 milligrams in ordinary eggs).

Fill Your Bread Bin

Whole-grain breads are great sources of a variety of important nutrients, including fiber and vitamin E. If your partner eats only white bread, buy a loaf of light wheat bread for him to try. It's refined, so many nutrients are lost, but it has the texture of white bread and one advantage over white and even whole grain breads: more fiber. Two slices of Wonder Light Wheat bread, for example, provide 6 grams of fiber. Two slices of whole wheat bread contain about 4 grams of fiber; two slices of white contain less than 1 gram.

Ideally, you and your partner should eat whole-grain bread. Don't be fooled by names like "seven-grain" or "multigrain." Such breads may well be made from a variety of grains, but unless they are specifically called "whole," those grains are processed. The milling process strips the bran and germ from the grain, removing about 40 different nutrients along with them. Sure, manufacturers enrich processed bread, but they add back only about eight of the lost nutrients. To find a loaf that is made from whole grain, check the ingredient list (near the nutrition label). The word "whole" should appear in front of whatever grain is listed. Most people who switch over to whole-grain breads soon find both the taste and texture so enjoyable that they'd never go back to the "enriched" but duller varieties.

A few more bread-buying tips: avoid croissants—they're high in fat. Look for whole-wheat varieties of French, Italian, and pita (pocket) breads. Whole-wheat tortillas are also available.

From the Store to the Table

Getting healthy foods into the house is half the battle. The other half involves learning how to present or prepare them in ways that are healthy and appealing to the eyes, the nose, and the palate. That will take some dedication on your part.

"At first, it was hard to get into the routine of using new foods and cooking techniques," says Marcia Shainis, whom we met at the beginning of this chapter. "I was frustrated," she continues. "I felt limited as to what I could make. It took some experimenting, but now we have a selection of healthy, low-fat staples that work for us."

Marcia recommends developing some dinner options that require a lot of preparation, some that require a little preparation, and some that require no preparation. "Don't feel guilty if you don't spend an hour in the kitchen every night. There are healthy things you can eat without slaving over the stove. If you make a big deal every night, you'll lose interest."

Marcia's most important resources are the Moosewood Restaurant's vegetarian cookbooks, Jane Brody's *Good Food Book*, and *Cooking Light* and *Vegetarian Times*

WHERE TO FIND THE "TOP 10" NUTRIENTS

This table highlights the dozen leading food sources of the 10 most important nutrients. Lower-fat foods are emphasized over foods high in fat, *even if a higher-fat food is a better source of a particular nutrient*. The foods are ranked highest to lowest, and the rankings are based on comparisons by weight. Try incorporating some of these foods into your family's diet.

BETA CARTENE

Beta carotene is an important antioxidant nutrient that may help protect against cancer. It's also converted by the body into vitamin A, necessary for maintaining healthy skin, teeth, mucous membranes, and skeletal and soft tissue, and for promoting good vision.

Carrots	Beet greens
Sweet potatoes	Spinach
Dandelion greens	Arugula
Turnip greens	Watercress
Kale	Hubbard squash
Butternut squash	Red bell peppers

VITAMIN C

Vitamin C's antioxidant properties may be useful in protecting against cancer and cataracts. In addition, it aids in iron absorption and in healing wounds.

Fuyu persimmon	Brussels sprouts
Red bell peppers	Cauliflower
Kale	Papaya
Kiwi fruit	Turnip greens
Broccoli	Strawberries
Arugula	Red cabbage

FOLACIN

Folacin (also called folate or folic acid) has been shown to be a potent factor in reducing certain birth defects and also may help protect against cervical cancer and heart disease. It acts with vitamin B_{12} to produce red blood cells.

Turnip greens	Romaine lettuce
Spinach	Asparagus
Mustard greens	Beets
Lentils	Okra
Pinto beans	Broccoli
Chickpeas	Artichokes

CALCIUM

Calcium's main function is to build and maintain strong bones and teeth, but it also plays a role in the regulation of heartbeat and other muscle contractions.

Part-skim mozzarella	Turnip greens
Arugula	Dandelion greens
Part-skim ricotta	Amaranth (a grainlike product)
Sardines (with bones)	Kale
Salmon (with bones)	Low-fat or skim milk
Low-fat plain yogurt	Watercress

IRON

Iron is crucial for the proper development of red blood cells. Women of childbearing age need to pay special attention to iron intake, since iron is lost monthly during menstruation.

Clams	Tofu
Quinoa (a grainlike product)	Oats
Lentils	Barley
Amaranth	Millet
Legumes (beans, soybeans, peanuts, chickpeas)	Beef
Oat bran	Whole-wheat bread

POTASSIUM

This mineral is important for muscle contractions and nerve impulses. There's some evidence that a high-potassium diet can help lower high blood pressure and reduce the risk of stroke.

Dried apricots	Chestnut
Raisins	Water chestnuts
Prunes	Halibut
Dried figs	Spinach
Trout	Beet greens
Clams	Fennel

ZINC

Zinc plays a major role in the proper functioning of the immune system, in tissue repair, and in the replication of DNA and RNA (the building blocks for our genes).

Oysters	Almonds
Pumpkin Seeds	Turkey, dark meat
Beef	Sunflower seeds
Pecans	Swiss cheese
Cashews	Goose
Lamb	Part-skim mozzarella

COMPLEX CARBOHYDRATES

Carbohydrates are the body's primary fuel, and foods high in complex carbohydrates are usually loaded with nutrients and fiber. (Vegetables such as potatoes, parsnips, and artichokes are also good sources.)

Barley	Triticale (a grain created by
Wheat	crossing wheat and rye)
Rice	Quinoa
Pasta	Oats
Buckwheat	Amaranth
Millet	Pinto beans
Rye	

FIBER

A diet high in fiber has been linked to the prevention or control of many diseases and disorders, including constipation, diverticulitis, diabetes, colon cancer, and heart disease.

Wheat-bran cereal	Barley
Pinto beans	Amaranth
Wheat	Sunchokes (the underground stem
Kidney beans	of a type of sunflower)
Triticale	Whole-wheat pasta
Great northern beans	Chickpeas
Oat bran	

PROTEIN

Protein supplies amino acids that the body needs to produce muscle tissue and carry out important enzymatic functions. Protein from animal sources often comes packed with fat. Below are protein sources that contain 4 grams or less of fat per 3.5-ounce serving.

Beef, top round, select cut	Rye
Chicken breast, no skin	Amaranth
Turkey breast, no skin	Wild Rice
Tuna, canned in water	Quinoa
Scallops	Cottage cheese
Legumes	Whole-wheat bread

Reprinted with permission from the *University of California at Berkeley Wellness Letter*, © Health Letter Associates, 1992. To order a one-year subscription, call 800–829–9170.

magazines. Her advice to women whose partners aren't open to dietary changes: "Try to stick with foods he likes, but modify how you prepare and cook them. If he's a meat-and-potatoes man, choose lower-fat cuts of meat and broil or barbecue the meat. Make low-fat mashed potatoes with skim milk. If your man likes bacon, ask him to try Canadian bacon—it has far less fat than the Anglo-American variety. Use an egg substitute to make scrambled eggs or pancakes. Sauté onion or garlic in wine or chicken broth instead of oil—he'll never know the difference."

Healthy cooking is easier now than it was 10 years ago because there are so many low fat products in the supermarket. "Some of those products are better than others," says Marcia. "You have to keep trying."

In addition to buying healthier foods and cooking by healthier methods, work on changing the role food plays in your life. For example, Pat Corbett and her family try not to link food with recreational activities. "If we go on a car trip or to the beach, I don't bring food," says Pat. "Food isn't the focus of our lives. We eat at mealtimes, then we move on to other activities."

Once you and your partner get used to the dietary changes you make, if you're like most folks who do the same thing, you won't look back. "I used to be a dairy freak," says Danny Shainis. "If I was at a party, you'd find me next to the cheese platter. Curtailing my dairy intake was the most difficult thing for me. It used to be I couldn't stand fat-free cheese, but it's tolerable to me now. As I've cut back on eating regular cheese, my taste has changed. In fact, if I have something now with a lot of real cheese on it, I feel sluggish afterwards."

Change is never easy. But it's almost always easier with a partner. Danny Shainis agrees: "The most fortunate thing for me is having a wife who takes my diet very seriously. She completely changed the way she cooks. I take it pretty seriously, too. Having had two heart attacks made me realize that a third one might be my last."

TWENTY-ONE TASTE-TESTED TIPS FOR A HEALTHIER KITCHEN

Simple changes in the way food is prepared and served can make meals a lot healthier. The tips that follow have been tested in real life; they come from the people whose stories appear within this book. You and your mate may not notice these changes and substitutions, but your bodies will.

1. Use a cooking spray instead of oil to grease baking pans. You also can use a cooking spray for frying.

2. If you're cooking with oil, use half the amount called for in the recipe. "If a dinner recipe calls for one tablespoon of oil, I use a half tablespoon," says Mary Regan. "We don't taste the difference, but if you're sautéing, you need to watch the pan a little more closely so foods don't stick." When frying, get the pan and oil very hot before adding food. The hotter the oil, the less time the food will have to be fried, and the less oil it will absorb.

3. Cook meat in cookware specifically designed for lower fat preparation of meat (available in better cookware stores).

4. Use a lot of herbs and spices. They can replace flavor lost when fat and salt are reduced. "Frequently, I use double the amount of herbs and spices called for," says Mary Regan. "We like the flavors they add."

5. To reduce the amount of damaging hydrogenated vegetable oil and saturated fat in baked goods, choose recipes that call for oil instead of margarine or butter.

6. Use a spray margarine substitute on baked potatoes, corn on the cob, and pancakes. It has no fat and no calories.

7. Use an egg substitute or egg whites instead of whole eggs. (Substitute two egg whites or ¼ cup of egg substitute for every whole egg.) Because all of an egg's fat and cholesterol are in the yolk, this strategy will help you reduce the artery-clogging potential of baked goods, pancakes, and egg dishes.

8. To make a lower-fat turkey gravy: make sure the turkey is done two hours ahead of time. Put the drippings in the freezer. When the fat has risen to the top, skim it off.

9. The same idea can be used for stews, soup stocks, and other dishes in which fat cooks into the liquid. Cook these dishes a day in advance so that they can be refrigerated until the fat hardens and rises to the top. Remove the fat with a spoon before serving.

10. When you want something simple to throw on the grill, try a tuna or salmon steak instead of beef.

11. Make a leaner burger. "I make our burgers with a fifty-fifty mixture of lean ground beef and ground turkey breast, to which I add a little onion," says Mary Regan. "It makes a pretty good burger!" Mary also uses ground turkey breast to make meat loaf.

12. Don't overcook red meat. Doing so on a routine basis can triple a person's risk of stomach cancer.

13. Broil, baste, or bake beef, pork, and poultry instead of pan-frying them.

14. When broiling, roasting, or baking, use a rack to allow fat to drain off.

15. Instead of basting with drippings, keep meat moist with fruit juices, wine, or an oil-based marinade (use canola or olive oil).

16. Make vegetarian chili. "It's very hearty," says Marcia Shainis. "No one will ever miss the ground beef."

17. Remove the skin from chicken or turkey before eating.

18. Steam vegetables rather than boiling them in water (valuable nutrients can be dissolved in—and be discarded with—the water).

19. Rinse canned beans before using to reduce the salt content.

20. Use low-fat or fat-free cheese. "We use fat-free cheeses," says John Regan. "Do I like them as well? No. But I've gotten used to them and I figure it's a sacrifice worth making for better health."

21. For snacking, buy low-fat or fat-free crackers and eat them with something other than cheese. Try hummus or a mixture of fat-free cottage cheese and red relish. Eat pretzels instead of potato chips, or try baked chips. (Tip: keep them in the freezer so they stay crisp.)

5

GET YOUR MAN MOVING

> *Health is the vital principle of bliss, and exercise, of health.*
>
> *James Thomson*

As we pointed out in the previous two chapters, most women have some measure of control over what food comes into the house and how it's prepared. There are healthy changes you can make in the kitchen that your partner won't even notice. The same isn't true of exercise. You can't sneak exercise in on your partner. He has to do it himself.

"With exercise, it's really simple," says Bill Heggie, a marketing strategist in Portland, Maine. "It's like the Nike tagline: 'Just do it.' You have to say that to yourself, often. Hearing it from someone else won't do the trick." If that's the case, why are we writing this chapter? Because, even though what Bill Heggie says is true, there are many things a woman can do to create a home environment that encourages a man to keep fit.

"I've heard over and over again that you can't change anyone," says Kathy Heggie, a project manager with a software company in Portland, Maine. "The first step for me was to express my feelings about the weight Bill has gained since we were married and to try to have a civil discussion about it. Once all had been said, I resigned myself to the fact that, ultimately, he's the one who needs to lose the weight. I counted my blessings, then began making sure that our house was generally filled with healthy food and encouraged Bill to join a health club."

Because Bill's schedule is hectic, Kathy encouraged him to join a club close to his office. The club is more expensive than others in Portland, but Kathy wanted to make it as easy as possible for Bill to work out. She knew, too, that the little luxuries the club offers would help Bill relax.

"After Bill joined the club," says Kathy, "he told me that he enjoys it more than any other club to which he has belonged. The pay off I get from seeing him pursue his goals and enjoying the process is much greater than the extra cost incurred."

Kathy worked with Bill to devise a schedule that would allow him the time he needed to work out routinely. (Although Bill is a bit of an early bird, the idea behind the schedule is one that other working couples with children could use.)

Here's how a typical day in the life of the Heggie family goes: Bill wakes at 4:00 A.M., does a little work, then drives to the gym. He's there at 5:30 A.M., and at work by 7:30 A.M. Kathy gets the couple's three children ready for day care and drops them off at the sitter's house on her way to work. At 4:30 P.M., when Bill's energy is flagging, he leaves work, picks up the children, brings them home, and feeds them dinner. That leaves Kathy free to work late or get to the gym herself.

The way the Heggies divide household responsibilities gives Bill the flexibility he needs to meet all of his work deadlines without giving up any workouts. For example, he's the family's "laundry marshal." While time consuming, washing laundry is a task that can be done at virtually any time of the day or night. Kathy, on the other hand, tends to daily chores like keeping the kitchen clean and tidying up after the children.

As with other areas of behavior, one of the most important things a woman can do to help her partner stick to a fitness routine is to set a good example. "My wife, Kathy, stays in shape herself," says Bill, whose goal is to lose 50 pounds. "When we go somewhere together, I'm aware of the contrast between us. That's part of what has motivated me to start working out again."

Fifteen Good Reasons to Be Active

Most people are aware that exercise is good for you. But a general awareness isn't usually enough to get someone up off the couch. Here are some specific facts that might convince your partner to start exercising or keep him committed to an active lifestyle.

1. Staying fit can increase the length of his life. Several studies show that active people are about 20 to 30 percent less likely to die of any cause at a given age than sedentary people. In fact, being sedentary increases a person's risk of dying prematurely as much as smoking one pack of cigarettes each day.

2. Vigorously active men have better sex. A study at the University of California, San Diego, compared previously inactive men who walked for one hour four times a week to men who participated in more strenuous forms of aerobic exercise. After nine months, the serious exercisers reported an increase in sexual desire, 30 percent more intercourse, more pleasure from orgasm, and fewer sex-related problems. The walkers reported no change in any of those areas.

3. Exercise increases the size and efficiency of the heart. This, in turn, lowers the heart rate (pulse), which reduces wear and tear on the coronary muscles. A strong heart also improves the body's ability to cope with and recover from injury and illness.

4. Exercise helps to reduce LDL ("bad") cholesterol and increase HDL ("good") cholesterol. Keeping cholesterol at healthy levels reduces risk of stroke and heart disease. According to a study at Yale, men who are inactive are nearly seven times more likely to suffer a stroke than men who are moderately or very active. Regular exercisers are 45 percent less likely to have a heart attack than non-exercisers.

5. Regular exercise appears to reduce risk of some cancers, including those of the colon and breast.

6. People who exercise are at reduced risk of osteoporosis. The bone-thinning disease is commonly thought of as a woman's illness, but it occurs quite frequently in men, too. Any weight-bearing exercise, such as walking or weight lifting, increases bone strength, which reduces the risk of osteoporosis-related fractures. That's important because in older adults a simple broken bone can cause complications that lead to disability and even death.

7. A sedentary lifestyle may be the primary cause of 30 to 50 percent of adult-onset diabetes cases. For those who have diabetes (type I or type II), exercise can help reduce long-term cardiovascular complications such as small blood vessel disease, diabetic retinopathy and heart disease.

8. Exercise boosts mood and self-confidence by releasing endorphins, chemicals in the brain that affect sensations of pain and emotions. In fact, researchers at Tufts University found that a weight-lifting program alleviated depression in 14 of 17 patients. Endorphins also increase sexual arousal for 60 to 90 minutes after 10 minutes or more of activity.

9. More than 150 studies confirm that exercise reduces the negative, internal effects of stress. It prompts the body to pump stress-managing endorphins into the bloodstream and decreases muscle tension.

10. Exercise significantly increases the likelihood that a person who loses weight will be able to keep it off. One way it helps is by decreasing appetite; another is by burning excess body fat.

11. Moderately intense physical activity, especially when done in the late afternoon, helps to relieve insomnia. Exercise is an especially good way to combat sleeplessness because it increases the amount of time the body spends in deep, restorative sleep.

12. Exercise can make the brain work better. Researchers believe that the improved mental function seen in subjects following strenuous exercise may be the result of increased flow of blood and memory-related chemicals to the brain.

13. Exercise improves reaction time. In a British study, people who walked for 20 minutes or more daily experienced significantly less age related deterioration in reaction time than those who walked less or not at all. That could translate into fewer accidents and falls for older adults.

14. Parents who exercise raise children who exercise. Only 22 percent of children are physically active for 30 minutes every day of the week. That's one of the reasons that one in five American children is overweight. When you consider that an overweight child has a higher chance of becoming an overweight adult (which will put him or her at increased risk for heart disease, diabetes, cancer, arthritis, and other diseases), the importance of starting healthy habits early becomes apparent.

15. If your man doesn't use it, he may lose it. Exercise enables men and women to remain more active as they get older by increasing muscle strength. Strong muscles allow greater mobility and fewer injuries than weak ones.

FOUR WAYS TO HELP YOUR CHILDREN ENJOY EXERCISE
According to the Centers for Disease Control and Prevention, children are more likely to be physically active if parents, schools, and communities follow these four pointers (each tip is followed by our suggestions for implementing that tip):

1. Emphasize enjoyable participation in physical activities that are easily done throughout life. Golf, tennis, walking, swimming, basketball, soccer, volleyball, softball—these are activities in which adults frequently participate. Sports such as football, field hockey, wrestling, rugby, and ice hockey are more difficult for adults to integrate into daily life. While school-age children shouldn't be discouraged from participating in sports that require lots of organization, they should be strongly encouraged to take up simpler sports, too.

2. Offer a diverse range of noncompetitive and competitive activities appropriate for different ages and abilities. In addition to signing Junior up for an organized soccer league, get in the habit of taking a family walk after dinner. Make raking leaves and shoveling snow family activities. If your daughter doesn't make the school basketball team, encourage her to keep playing socially by putting up a hoop in the driveway and shooting baskets together.

3. Give young people the skills and confidence they need to be physically active. This can be done in many fun ways. Choose several that appeal to you and your children. For example: kick a soccer ball around; hit a tennis ball against a wall; dribble a basketball; shoot baskets; throw and catch a ball; hit a ball with a bat; try to keep a beach ball up in the air as long as possible; chase each other around the yard; play leap frog; or do somersaults.

4. Set rules that prompt activity and limit inactivity. For example, limit time spent watching television, using a computer, or playing video games. Require that children take turns walking the dog. Don't drive children to their friends' houses if walking or riding a bicycle is a safe alternative.

Exercising with Disabilities

People with disabilities stand to benefit from exercise as much as—if not more than—people without disabilities. In addition to reducing risk of heart disease, high blood pressure, colon cancer, and diabetes, exercise can help people with disabling conditions improve their stamina and muscle strength. By reducing symptoms of anxiety and depression, exercise can promote general feelings of well-being in people living with a chronic illness.

In the Surgeon General's report on physical activity and health, experts send these key messages to people with disabilities:

• Physical activity need not be strenuous to achieve health benefits.

• Significant health benefits can be obtained with a moderate amount of physical activity, preferably daily. The same moderate amount of activity can be obtained in longer sessions of moderately intense activities (such as 30 to 40 minutes of wheeling oneself in a wheelchair) or in shorter sessions of more strenuous activities (such as 20 minutes of wheelchair basketball).

• Additional health benefits can be gained through greater amounts of physical activity. People who can maintain a regular routine of physical activity that is of longer duration or of greater intensity are likely to derive greater benefit.

• People with disabilities should first consult a physician before beginning a program of physical activity to which they are unaccustomed.

• Social support from family and friends has been consistently and positively related to regular physical activity.

FITNESS WEB SITES FOR THE DISABLED
Internet resources for disabled fitness enthusiasts include:
• **SportsQuest**: http://www.sportsquest.com. Click on the bar that says "disabled" to find a list of useful Internet sites, indexed by sport. This extensive list of links covers 29 sports.
• **National Sports Center for the Disabled:** http://www.nscd.org/nscd. The NSCD is a nonprofit organization that provides recreation for children and adults with disabilities. Programs are offered in white-water rafting, hiking, sailing, snow skiing, and in-line skating.
• **U.S. Association of Blind Athletes:** http://www.usaba.org. The USABA is an amateur organization that provides sport opportunities at the state, regional, national, and international levels. The Web site provides descriptions and contact names for several sports, including alpine skiing, athletics, goalball, judo, Nordic skiing, powerlifting, and swimming.
• **International Paralympic Committee:** http://info.lut.ac.uk/research/paad/ipc/ipc.html. The Paralympics are the Olympic games for the physically disabled. In addition to information about the Games, this site provides links to sport and disability Web sites.

What Motivates Men to Exercise?

While women, in general, exercise in order to look or feel better, many men are motivated by challenge and competition. "With things going well at work and at home, I needed a new challenge to focus on," says Bill. Another man we interviewed said that seeing his neighbor trim down and shape up spawned competitive feelings that urged him to begin his own exercise program.

Understanding what turns your man on, so to speak, will allow you to help him pick an exercise routine that suits his needs. If he needs a competitive outlet, for example, he might enjoy getting his exercise by playing games. Whether he chooses racquetball, basketball, volleyball, golf, or some other sport will depend on his personal preferences and experience. You can help by calling the town's recreation office to find out what leagues exist in your area and who your partner can call to find out more about them.

If your partner prefers to compete with himself, he might try running, swimming, biking, walking, hiking, or weight training. Again, you can make it easier for your man to get started by doing some legwork for him. Pick up local trail maps at the library. Check the local paper for notices of biking clubs. Ask your acquaintances about their favorite running routes. Make preliminary phone calls to local gyms to ask about facilities and membership prices. Then tour the most promising ones with your mate.

Be a Fitness Buddy

What else can you do to help? "One of the best ways women can help men get healthy is to try to really engage men in their fitness activities," says Michael Lafavore, editor-in-chief of *Men's Health* magazine. "If a woman is a runner, she should try to interest her partner in running with her. That approach works far better than assigning a chore, as in: 'You need to go running to lose weight.'"

A 1996 survey commissioned by the President's Council on Physical Fitness and Sports supports Lafavore's theory. Respondents said that having a friend or relative to work out with was the most effective encouragement to start exercising and stay with it.

That approach has worked for Sheila Beahm, the airline pilot we met in Chapter 2. She asked her husband, Larry Schuermann, to join her for a yoga session, and now he joins her on a regular basis. In other instances, Sheila uses a more subtle approach. For example, she has a workout video that includes aerobics and exercises done with weights. "I never say, 'Hey honey, let's do the video,' " says Sheila. "I just do it when he's around the house and let him slip into the routine."

When Michelle Bromley started to exercise, her fiancé, Roman LePree, took notice. "He saw me lose weight and thought he might try it. Now we work out every day, and I've become a certified personal trainer. We went from sleeping 12 hours a night to being at the gym at 6 A.M. and working out for an hour every morning. The nice thing about being committed to exercise together is that when the alarm goes off, I don't feel like I'm the only one getting up."

In addition to working out in a gym, between them Michelle and Roman play basketball, volleyball, football, golf, tennis, and baseball. They don't play all those sports together, and they don't play all of them on a regular basis. But they do make activity part of their daily lives.

Each partner is inspired by the other's active lifestyle. In addition, says Michelle: "When one of us gets bored of our routine, we just come up with a new sport to try together. It might be racquetball or jumping rope. We just get the stuff and try it."

Being active helps couples bond. "We do so many things

together," says Sheila. "We're into rock climbing, backpacking, white-water kayaking, rafting, and snow skiing, among other things. Larry is teaching me to windsurf, and I turned him on to open-ocean kayaking. We plan to get certified in scuba diving, which is new to both of us. Doing all these things is a big part of the glue that holds us together." Larry agrees, saying: "It's more fun doing things with someone you care about."

Not every couple can live a lifestyle that includes such a wide variety of exciting activities, but there are many sports that can be done just about anywhere by couples. Some examples are walking, biking, in-line skating, working out at a gym, shooting hoops in the driveway or at a local school, playing tennis on public courts, swimming, hiking, ice skating, and running.

 FITNESS WEB SITES WORTH VISITING
If your man is into the Internet, he may enjoy visiting these sites:

• **The American Council on Exercise:** http://www.acefitness.org. ACE certifies fitness professionals and promotes the benefits of an active lifestyle to the public. The site includes informative fitness articles and links to other fitness and health sites.

• **The Internet's Fitness Resource:** http://www.netsweat.com. In addition to fitness information and advice, this site offers an extensive collection of links to other fitness sites. These include sport-specific sites and sites dedicated to the topic of children and fitness.

How Much Exercise Is Enough?

To achieve a minimum level of physical fitness that will provide general health benefits and help in weight management, the American College of Sports Medicine and the U.S. Public Health Service recommend 30 minutes of moderate aerobic activity each day. Aerobic activities are those that involve continuous motion and require your heart and lungs to work harder to supply your cells with more oxygen. By improving the health of those vital organs, aerobic workouts lead to improvements in overall condition and endurance.

Moderate activity for 30 minutes a day is enough to burn 150 calories a day or just over 1,000 calories a week. According to the Surgeon General's Report on Physical Activity and Health, examples of moderate activity that burn about 150 calories per episode include:

- Brisk walking for 35 minutes
- Bicycling 4 miles in 15 minutes
- Stair-walking for 15 minutes
- Playing volleyball for 45 minutes
- Washing windows or floors for 45 to 60 minutes
- Gardening for 45 minutes
- Dancing fast for 30 minutes
- Washing and waxing a car for 45 to 60 minutes
- Raking leaves for 30 minutes
- Shoveling snow for 20 minutes
- Chopping wood for 30 minutes
- Engaging in sexual activity for 30 minutes

The American Heart Association basically agrees with these guidelines for the promotion of improved general health levels. It recommends that adults take three or four brisk 30-minute walks each week. In addition, the AHA recommends small habit changes that can increase daily activity. For example, routinely take the stairs instead of the elevator, and choose the parking spot farthest from the door wherever you go.

However, when addressing the issue of preventing heart disease and other serious health problems such as diabetes, researchers have found that the more a person exercises, the more he or she reduces personal health risks. For example, studies show that burning 1,500 to 2,000 calories per week in physical exercise (about 40 minutes of brisk walking every day) may lower a person's risk of adult-onset diabetes by as much as 25 percent.

One advantage of more strenuous exercise is that it's the only way to boost aerobic capacity (heart and lung functional capability). Why is aerobic capacity important? For one thing, risk of death declines as aerobic fitness increases. Another reason your man might want to boost aerobic fitness is better sex. One study at the University of California, San Diego, found a direct correlation between aerobic fitness and sexual performance (defined in the study as lasting longer and having more orgasms).

So how much exercise is enough? The answer is simple enough. If your partner is currently sedentary, working up to the ACSM/USPHS recommended level of activity would be an excellent first goal. Once he gets used to being active and starts to feel more energetic, he may want to move up to the next level, regularly engaging in more intense aerobic exercise. However, even if he never moves beyond 30 minutes of moderate activity daily, he'll be a lot healthier than he was when sedentary.

If your man has favorite hobbies that don't burn much energy, help him find ways to increase the activity level of those hobbies. For example, if he likes golf, encourage him to walk the course instead of riding in a cart (if the club allows walking). If he's an angler, suggest that he hike to his favorite fishing hole. If he loves music, sign yourselves up for a dancing class.

If the man in your life is already active on a daily basis, encourage him to step it up a level by taking on a new activity. For example, he might try weight training, swimming, or a sport you can take up together, like bicycling or tennis.

Help Your Man to a Sensible Start

The structure of an exercise routine deserves more attention than most people give it. Setting goals that are reasonable for the person exercising is the key—anything too ambitious may discourage a would-be exerciser from sticking to his plan. Starting up slowly is important, too, because too much exertion too soon can lead to injuries that force the exerciser to take a break from his program. An injury break early in an exercise regimen—before the new athlete has experienced the psychological benefits of exercise—can easily become a permanent break.

A man whose most strenuous daily activity has been getting out of bed might want to start with 10 minutes of walking three times a week. He can work up to a goal of two 10-minute walks each day. Not only is 20 minutes of walking an achievable goal, breaking it into two 10-minute segments increases the likelihood that your man will stick to his program. One study showed that walkers who broke their daily exercise into 10-minute segments actually wound up walking more than they set out to. Those exercisers who took one long walk each day ended up falling short of their goals.

Two 10-minute walks may sound like sissy stuff to your partner. Emphasize that starting this way will increase the likelihood that he'll stick to his program. He can increase the intensity of his program once the walks have become habit and he has started to feel some benefit from them.

Changing daily habits to include exercise is critical to your man's success. Walking is something that doesn't require instruction or equipment—distractions that might take your partner's focus off his primary task of making exercise an integral part of his life. There will be plenty of time later to try new sports and more strenuous workouts.

One of the keys to becoming more active—permanently—is to build slowly on a series of small successes. That strategy helps exercisers to avoid frustration and injuries. It also can save you a lot of money. Most of us have at some point in our lives purchased exercise equipment or a health-club membership card. Too often, that thing we thought would magically prompt us to become active doesn't see the light of day after a week or two. Starting his new exercise program with walking, or any other activity that can be done free of charge, will give your partner a chance to get into the habit of exercising before he spends a lot of money.

DON'T GET GYPPED BY A GYM

Before joining a gym, send for a copy of "How To Choose a Quality Fitness Facility" from the International Association of Fitness Professionals. It explains what to look for in a health club. Some examples it cites are a health screening, a trial period, and a free equipment demonstration. Also look for a facility that offers a variety of activities to help keep boredom at bay. To receive a copy of the booklet, send a self-addressed, stamped envelope to the International Association of Fitness Professionals, 6190 Cornerstone Ct. E., Suite 204, San Diego, CA 92121.

Make a Plan

Help your partner establish a routine that includes exercise at least three days each week. Sit down with him and help him plan how he'll work exercise sessions into his schedule. Perhaps you'll pick the children up from day care on workout days or get them ready for school in the morning while he heads for the gym. And don't forget to ask your partner to pitch in so you can exercise, too. Maybe he'll do the grocery shopping on Saturday morning or bring your son to Boy Scouts so you can scoot out to the gym.

One important note: if your man is over 35 and has been inactive for several years, is a smoker, or has a history of heart disease, high blood pressure, high cholesterol, diabetes, or another serious illness, he should check with his doctor before beginning an exercise program.

The less you and your partner have to plan and decide on a daily basis, the less likely either of you is to decide the whole thing isn't worth the trouble. A systematic approach is sure to help make exercise a matter of habit. Those who think of exercise as being as much a part of their life as brushing their teeth or going to work are the most likely to become habitual exercisers.

TEN WAYS TO GET YOUR MAN MOVING

1. Make music. When men in a Massachusetts study were asked to ride a stationary bike until they were exhausted, those who listened to music rode 29 percent longer. Make a tape of your man's favorite tunes (from CDs or tapes that you own or have borrowed). If he doesn't already own a personal tape player, buy him one. Then give him the gift of music to move by.

2. Practice what you preach. You can't advise your man to get moving if your own idea of a workout is unloading the dishwasher. Your words will ring hollow unless you're committed to an exercise program—even if it's simply walking 20 minutes a day. Try working out together, at least some days. People who work out in pairs tend to stick with their routines longer than those who exercise solo.

3. Don't use fear as a motivator. Even if it works in the short term, telling your husband that he's a heart attack waiting to happen is unlikely to result in a long-term commitment to exercise. Once his fear dissipates, which it will, so will his reason to work out.

4. Do use self-esteem as a motivator. Over time, internal rewards are better motivators than external rewards. Emphasize the improvements that exercise can make in how your man *feels* (stronger, a greater sense of control over his life, more energetic) over weight loss or other external factors. Tell your partner how exercise has improved your self-image and confidence. Talk about how good your workouts makes you feel.

5. Help your partner identify—then replace—negative beliefs. Ask him what he considers to be the biggest barrier to his exercising on a regular basis. Then help him replace that belief with a positive thought. For example, let's say your partner feels he's just too out of shape to exercise. He's doesn't want to work out at a health club because he'll be embarrassed by his lack of strength and stamina. Remind him that he has been in good shape at other times in his life. Suggest that he start walking with you in the mornings and exercising with handheld weights while he watches the evening news. Then when he's in better shape, he can join a gym.

6. Help your partner identify his own primary motivators. What's important to your partner? Does he want to avoid taking medication for his borderline high blood pressure or unhealthy cholesterol level? Does he want more energy and increased cardiovascular endurance? Does he want to sleep better at night? Is he looking for enhanced self-esteem, improved appearance, or a release from stress? Exercise can provide all those benefits. Once your partner has identified what's most important to him, he can focus on those goals as his primary motivators. He can structure his routine to best suit his goals and measure his progress in ways that are most meaningful to him.

For example, if your partner is most concerned about improving his ability to manage stress, he might plan to exercise after work. That way, he can burn off some of the day's negative or hostile feelings, and come home more relaxed. You, in turn, will know to frame your compliments and encouraging words in terms of how he's handling stress. You might say, "Gee, honey, you've been so patient with the children while they're getting ready for bed. It's nice to see you enjoying your time with them." If your man is most concerned about his cardiovascular health, he can focus on aerobic exercise rather than weight lifting. You can emphasize the benefits of his improved stamina and any positive effects exercise has had on his blood pressure and cholesterol level.

7. Help your partner identify his ideal exercise environment. For some people, time outdoors is one of the biggest benefits of exercise. Others enjoy the social aspects of exercising at a health club. Still others are most comfortable in the privacy of their own home. Convenience should also play a role in decisions about where to work out. If the health club is twenty minutes away, will it really be feasible to get there on a regular basis? Talk to your partner about the pros and cons of various exercise environments to help him identify which appeals most to him. Choosing the right environment improves the odds that a person will stick to a fitness routine.

8. Encourage your man to build variety into his exercise program. Variety will help him remain committed to exercise by preventing boredom.

9. Help your partner find activities he enjoys. Some people can't abide walking on a treadmill; others love to grab a magazine and walk miles to nowhere. Swimming suits some people; others think it's all wet. Some people love the social aspects of an aerobics class; others feel self-conscious and out of place. Your man is much more likely to stick with exercise if he chooses an activity he actually enjoys. Exercise shouldn't be drudgery. It should be fun—at least most of the time.

10. Make fitness a part of your lives. People are more likely to remain active if they incorporate exercise into their lives. In other words, exercise shouldn't be something you have to do three times a week or that you do only at the health club. Think of yourselves as active people. Make plans to take a hike, ride your bikes, or play tennis on the weekends. Encourage your partner to join in a Saturday game of pickup basketball. Play volleyball when you're at the beach. Walk instead of taking the subway when you're in the city.

6

PROTECT REPRODUCTIVE AND SEXUAL HEALTH

A little neglect may breed mischief: for want of a nail the shoe was lost; for want of a shoe the horse was lost, and for want of a horse the rider was lost.

Benjamin Franklin

Most men are at least aware that there are things they can do to keep their hearts healthy, but chances are your mate hasn't given a second thought to maintaining his reproductive and sexual health. That's a shame, because diseases of the reproductive organs can be emotionally as well as physically devastating.

In this chapter, we'll look at what you can do to help your man avoid such problems as infertility and prostate disease, including cancer. We'll also discuss impotence and the advantages of male versus female sterilization for birth control.

First, here are 22 ways a man can reduce his general risk of reproductive and sexual health problems:

1. Eat a diet low in saturated fat and cholesterol.
Just as a high-fat diet can clog coronary arteries and reduce

blood flow to the heart, it can reduce blood flow to the penis. When blood flow to the penis is impeded, it becomes more difficult to achieve an erection. This phenomena has been called a "penis attack." Although this potential side effect is rarely emphasized when talk turns to the perils of fatty foods, men should be aware that a high-fat diet could render them impotent as they get older.

Eating a diet rich in fatty foods also may increase a man's risk of prostate cancer. A National Cancer Institute study found that men produced less of the male hormone testosterone when they consumed a low-fat (less than 20 percent of daily calories), high-fiber diet than they did when they followed a high-fat (41 percent fat), low-fiber diet. Because abnormally high testosterone levels are suspected of playing a role in the development of prostate cancer, experts suggest that eating a low-fat, high-fiber diet may help to ward off the disease.

As we have noted, diets low in fat have also been linked to reduced incidences of high blood pressure, heart disease, and diabetes—all of which increase a man's risk of impotence (in addition, of course, to the more serious risks of those diseases, which include disability and death).

2. Eat lots of fruits and vegetables. In a study of about 15,000 male doctors, those who had the largest amounts of beta carotene in their blood were less likely to develop prostate cancer than those who had the smallest amounts. Beta carotene is found in fruits and vegetables, especially those that are orange or red, including pumpkin, sweet potatoes, carrots, apricots, winter squash, tomatoes, and watermelon. Most experts recommend not taking beta carotene supplements because some studies have shown them to be ineffective and even dangerous.

Consuming a variety of fruits and vegetables will also

ensure that your man gets plenty of vitamin C, which is important to normal sperm production. Low vitamin C levels may also make sperm clump together, which can cause infertility. In addition to eating lots of vitamin-C-rich foods, your man may want to consider taking a supplement so that his daily intake falls between 200 milligrams and 1,000 milligrams.

3. Make sure to get enough zinc. Zinc plays an important role in the production of testosterone, the primary male hormone. Low levels can reduce sperm count and sperm motility (their ability to wriggle through a woman's reproductive tract to get to the egg), causing infertility. Those most at risk of not getting enough zinc are vegetarians who eat no animal products at all. Most experts don't recommend taking zinc supplements because too much zinc can interfere with copper absorption. Foods high in zinc include beef, lamb, seafood, egg yolk, milk, wheat germ, whole grains, and soybeans. The recommended daily allowance for zinc is 15 milligrams.

4. Eat plenty of tomato-based sauces. Tomatoes are rich in the antioxidant lycopene, which appears to help prevent prostate cancer. Fat helps move lycopene into the bloodstream, so choose foods like pizza and pasta with sauces that contain a little olive oil or canola oil. Why olive or canola? Because the fat they contain is monounsaturated, a type of fat that reduces artery-clogging LDL cholesterol while keeping artery-cleaning HDL cholesterol high.

5. Drink plenty of water. Water dilutes urine, making it less likely to irritate the prostate.

6. Go organic. In a Danish study, farmers whose diets included at least 25 percent organically grown fruits and vegetables produced 43 percent more sperm per milliliter of semen than other workers who didn't eat organic produce.

7. Maintain a healthy weight. Body fat affects hormone levels, which in turn, affect fertility. Obese men may have low levels of testosterone and high levels of estrogen, a combination that impedes sperm production. One more reason not to pig out—Swedish researchers found that men who admitted to frequent overeating were four times as likely to develop prostate cancer as those who said they did not routinely overeat.

8. Refrain from smoking cigarettes. Smoking appears to be a significant risk factor for penile cancer. In addition, smoking is linked to low sperm counts and sluggish sperm motility. Some studies suggest an increased risk of miscarriage when the male partner smokes. Last but by no means least, one expert estimates that tobacco use is responsible for 50 percent of impotence cases. (Cigarettes do their damage by impairing circulation of blood to the penis.)

9. Don't smoke pot. Regular, long-term use of marijuana decreases a man's sperm count and results in sperm abnormalities. In addition, researchers have found that THC, the active ingredient in marijuana, prevents mouse embryos from implanting in the uterus wall, which makes it impossible for a fetus to develop. Marijuana may have a similar effect on human reproduction.

10. Avoid excessive consumption of alcohol. Alcohol abuse plays havoc with the male reproductive system, reducing a man's ability to produce normal sperm cells. It also reduces testosterone levels and can cause impotence. As Shakespeare wisely pointed out in *Macbeth,* drinking alcohol "provokes the desire, but it takes away from the performance."

11. Don't take steroids. Most women enjoy a well-muscled man—but not at the high costs associated with the use of anabolic steroids. Men who use steroids on a regular basis are at increased risk for heart attack, stroke, liver disease, decreased testicle size, and low sperm count.

12. Use a condom if yours is not a monogamous relationship. Using a latex condom along with the spermicide nonoxynol-9 is the most effective way this side of abstinence to prevent STDs. In addition to reducing the wearer's risk of HIV, the virus that causes AIDS, the combination of condoms and nonoxynol-9 reduces the risk of contacting human papillomavirus (HPV), which is linked to penile cancer, and the herpes simplex virus type 2.

WHO SHOULD GET SNIPPED?

When you get tired of birth control pills, sponges, diaphragms, temperature tracking, and condoms, what do you do? If you're like many couples, you consider sterilization. For couples who aren't planning to have any more children, choosing sterilization is easy. Deciding who gets sterilized isn't.

"I've shouldered my share of reproductive responsibility by spending more than two years of my life pregnant, then enduring three turns at labor and delivery," says Christy. "Now it's Matt's turn. Besides, vasectomy is easier to do, cheaper, and less risky than tubal ligation."

Tubal ligation is the surgical procedure done to seal or cut the fallopian tubes so that eggs can no longer travel down from the ovaries to meet sperm. In vasectomy, the tubes that carry sperm from the testicles to the urethra, called the vas deferentia, are cut and sealed. This prevents sperm from becoming part of the semen that's ejaculated during intercourse. Neither procedure has a high complication rate. However, bear in mind that the fatality rate for tubal ligation is 3.5 per 100,000—compared to zero for vasectomy.

Vasectomy is easier to reverse than tubal ligation, although couples choosing either form of sterilization should consider it a permanent decision. Recent advances in microsurgical techniques, instruments, and suture materials have boosted vasectomy-reversal success rates to somewhere between 87 and 97 percent. About 50 percent of those couples subsequently achieve pregnancy.

So why do so many men, like Christy's husband Matt, get hung up about vasectomy? "Mostly," says Matt, "it's the procedure. Having to go to the doctor's office is bad enough, but the whole idea of someone messing with your testicles is really disturbing. Also, there's a subconscious fear that the procedure takes something away from you—your manhood, maybe."

To reassure your man, share these facts with him:

• Today's no-scalpel vasectomies take about ten minutes and are done in a doctor's office. As the name indicates, there's no incision and no stitches. After a local anesthetic is administered, a single puncture hole is made in the scrotum, about one-tenth of an inch in size (compared to the two half-inch incisions used in traditional vasectomy). The vas deferentia are pulled out, cut, and returned to the scrotum. The risk of post-procedure bleeding is less than 1 percent; the risk of infection is virtually zero.

• Vasectomy closes off the vas deferentia, which prevents sperm from joining the other fluids that make up semen. There's no noticeable change in the man's semen, because sperm make up no more than 5 percent of seminal fluid.

• Vasectomy has no physical effect on a man's virility because it doesn't interfere with the production of the male hormone testosterone. Your partner's sex drive, potency, male characteristics, and sexual pleasure should be unchanged. In fact, about 30 percent of men report enjoying sex more after vasectomy—probably because they no longer have to worry about pregnancy.

• Although one study found that men who had had a vasectomy were at increased risk for prostate cancer, subsequent studies have shown no increased incidence of prostate cancer following the procedure. A panel of experts convened by the National Institutes of Health concluded that there's no convincing evidence of a link between male sterilization and prostate cancer.

If your man agrees to a vasectomy, plan to pamper him for a couple of days following the procedure. He should rest and keep his feet up to reduce the risk of swelling and discomfort in his testicles. Buy him a postprocedure present: the latest book by his favorite author; a new CD; or a prepaid phone card so he can sit and catch up with old friends. Cook his favorite dinner and rent a movie he's been wanting to see. But before you turn to the tube, be sure to turn to your man and say, "Thanks, babe."

13. Wear a cup. Only 10 percent of men who participate in recreational sports wear an athletic cup or supporter. The other 90 percent are putting themselves at risk of an injury that, in addition to being extremely painful, could cause impotence or impair fertility.

When they do injure the family jewels, most men don't bother to see a doctor. In one study of 30 men whose testicles were injured severely enough to cause pain for at least 24 hours, as well as significant swelling and/or a broken blood vessel or blood clot, only one saw a physician at the time of the injury.

When the testicles take a blow from a ball, a kick, or anything else, swelling can reduce the flow of blood to the area and cause tissue death, which in turn can lead to scarring and a lowering of sperm production. A man who has taken a blow to the testicles should seek medical attention within four to six hours to help prevent long term adverse effects.

14. Treat erections with respect. An erect penis isn't as hardy as it looks. In fact, one expert estimates that three to four million men in the United States are impotent because of an injury to the penis that occurred during masturbation or intercourse. Men should always alert their partners if they feel any discomfort at all during sex. Experts advise that men grin and bear an erection that occurs at an inopportune time. Trying to get rid of it by holding or slapping it down or forcing it into jeans could cause injury.

An injury to an erect penis can leave scar tissue that may lead to Peyronie's disease, an unnatural bending or narrowing of the penis. Peyronie's disease can make intercourse virtually impossible. Fortunately, medical treatment usually alleviates the symptoms.

Many people aren't aware that an erect penis can be fractured. If you could look inside an erect penis, you would see two long, narrow chambers. These balloonlike chambers are called erectile bodies. When the penis is erect, the chambers are filled with blood. When an erect penis suffers blunt trauma (for example, when it hits a partner's pubic bone instead of the intended destination during intercourse), blood, which has no way of escaping from the erect penis, is forced suddenly into one area. The resulting pressure can cause the fluid to burst through the elastic covering of the erectile bodies (called the tunica). The erectile tissue is, literally, broken. Fracture is accompanied by a loud snapping sound, and is followed by bruising, swelling, and severe pain. A man who has noticed any of those symptoms should see a doctor as soon as possible. Penile fracture isn't an injury that takes care of itself. It requires immediate medical attention.

15. Modify your bicycle. Frequent bike riding can inflame the prostate, a small, doughnut-shaped gland that surrounds the urethra (the tube that carries urine out of the body). This makes it more difficult for a man to empty his bladder, which in turn increases the risk of a bladder infection. Prostate inflammation is most likely when cycling is done on a bike with a narrow, hard seat. Experts recommend using a softer, wider seat and pitching the seat forward slightly so that the weight of the body isn't putting pressure on the external reproductive organs. Raising the handlebars helps the rider feel that he's not going to slide off the bike.

16. Avoid tight underwear and tight pants—at least until you've completed your family. The jury is still out on this one, but several studies have found that wearing tight underwear raises sperm temperature, which can reduce the amount and quality of sperm. One French study found that the fertility of would-be fathers was reduced if their jobs exposed them to a hot work environment—for example, a job such as welding or one that requires lots of driving.

On the other hand, when researchers at Los Angeles Medical Center conducted a study to determine whether increasing the temperature of the scrotum could be used as a method of male birth control, they found that it couldn't. The study included 21 men who wore polyester-lined athletic supports throughout the day, every day, for one year. The result? Scrotal temperature was raised, but the increase didn't affect semen volume, sperm concentration, or sperm motility and morphology.

Despite the controversy, if you and your mate are trying to conceive, he may want to wear boxers instead of briefs. Likewise, he may want to avoid habitual use of hot tubs and saunas, which also increase scrotal temperature. These changes are simple enough to make, so why not be on the safe side?

RELATED WEB SITES

For more information on men's reproductive health issues, try these Internet sites:

• **Prostate Health:** http://www.prostatehealth.com. Run by the American Foundation for Urologic Disease, this site offers information on prostatitis, benign prostatic hyperplasia (BPH), and prostate cancer. It includes an international registry for men with BPH and an area where you can ask questions about BPH and its treatment.

- **Online Guide to Impotence:** http://www.impotent.com. This site includes information about impotence and its treatments as well as physician referrals. It's maintained by Pharmacia & Upjohn, the pharmaceutical company that markets the impotence drug Caverject.

- **Male Factor Infertility:** http://www.ivf.com/male.html. Everything you ever wanted to know about semen is included in this site, along with information about male reproductive physiology, assessment of male infertility, and artificial insemination. It's maintained by the Atlanta Reproductive Health Centre.

- **The Male Health Center:** http://www.malehealthcenter.com. This site features current, straightforward information on male reproductive health issues, men's preventive screenings, and sex.

17. Take stress seriously. Poorly managed stress can reduce semen quality and contribute to impotence. It also can aggravate the prostate gland, setting off prostatitis (an infection of the prostate). To learn what you can do to help your partner better handle stress, see Chapter 9, "Give Stress the Slip."

18. Urinate often. When men urinate infrequently, concentrated urine may get forced into the prostatic ducts during physical exertion. Once there, it's likely to cause prostatitis, a painful infection of the prostate that engenders fever, chills, body aches, and pain in the prostate (felt in the lower back and around the anus). Often, the infection in the prostate spreads to the nearby bladder, giving rise to additional symptoms that include frequent urination, an uncontrollable urge to urinate, and burning on urination. Men who have suffered through prostatitis would probably agree that it's well worth a man's time to heed the urge to

urinate rather than to hold it in until the end of the meeting, the end of a meal, or the end of a football game.

19. Don't over use decongestants. Although fine for
a severe cold, decongestants shouldn't be used habitually
at the first sign of a sniffle. They can tighten the prostate,
making it more difficult for urine to flow.

20. Follow prostate-cancer screening guidelines.
The American Cancer Society recommends that men aged
50 years or older should have a digital rectal exam (DRE)
and a prostate-specific antigen (PSA) blood test every year.
The ACS further advises that men who are at high risk of
prostate cancer—African-American men and men with a
family history of the disease—should begin annual screening at the age of 40. But some experts dispute the value
of routine PSA screening because there's no evidence that
the test reduces prostate-cancer morbidity or mortality. (For
more on prostate-cancer screenings, see Chapter 2, "Share
the Word on Screening.")

21. Perform a testicular self-exam once a month.
While there's no known way to prevent testicular cancer,
tumors that are found early can almost always be treated
successfully. Performing a testicular self-exam every month
greatly increases the odds that a tumor will be detected
early. Here's how to do it:

During or just after a warm shower (when the skin of
the scrotum is loose and relaxed), examine the testicles
one at a time. Roll the testicle between the thumb and
fingers. It should feel like a hard-boiled egg. Feel for any
lumps on the surface of the testicle, and notice if the testicle is hard or feels different in any other way from the last
exam. The two testicles shouldn't vary in size by more than
one-quarter inch, and each should be about one-and-a-half
inches across. Notice whether the testicle is enlarged or

differs in appearance in any way from the previous exam. Also look for unusual growths on the surface of the penis or under the skin. Such growths can be cancerous and should be evaluated by a physician.

Testicular cancer is most common among men between the ages of 15 and 35. However, older men aren't immune and should continue to do a monthly exam. The average age at which men with penile cancer are diagnosed is 58, but much younger men have been affected. The bottom line is a recommendation most men won't find too taxing (if your partner does, you might offer to help): all males should begin examining their external genitals in high school and should make it a lifelong habit.

22. Have sex—often. Finally, a recommendation that men are usually more than happy to embrace. Frequent ejaculations help empty the prostate of secretions that can cause or aggravate prostate problems. Sex helps reduce stress and boosts testosterone levels, both of which enhance fertility. Last, but not least, sex helps keep relationships going. Levels of oxytocin—sometimes called the bonding hormone—are boosted slightly whenever a person is touched. When he (or she) has enough close personal contact to bring on orgasm, oxytocin levels blast off, triggering feelings of love and tenderness. How often is often enough to reap all these benefits? Experts suggest aiming to have intercourse one to three times a week.

Reproductive health issues can be divided into two areas of concern: fertility and disease prevention. Fortunately, aiming for improved health in one area is likely to help achieve benefits in the other. For example, let's say you and your partner are thinking of starting a family and decide that he's going to quit smoking to boost fertility and to give your baby the best start possible. By accomplishing

that goal, he'll also be reducing his risk of prostate cancer—and lung cancer, too, of course.

Fighting Infertility with Lifestyle Changes

During seven years of infertility, Will and Sallie made several lifestyle changes to improve their odds of conceiving.
When it became clear that they had a fertility problem, the
first thing to go were Will's briefs. After the switch to boxers, however, two years of medical treatment passed before
the couple decided to take any additional steps.

At that point, Sallie told Will, who was smoking marijuana on a daily basis, that she wouldn't continue with
hormone injections and other medical interventions unless
he quit. "I wasn't going to try to have a baby anymore if
he was going to sabotage our efforts by smoking marijuana," says Sallie.

At first, Will just cut back. "I would quit just before each
cycle of intrauterine insemination was to begin, then smoke
again once we reached the point where conception would
have occurred if it were going to," he says. (Intrauterine
insemination, or IUI, is a fertility treatment in which sperm
are deposited directly into the uterus, bypassing the cervix.)

Sallie became pregnant twice with IUI. Sadly, both pregnancies ended in miscarriage. After the second miscarriage,
Will gave up marijuana completely. "There was no conversation about it," says Sallie. "It was real obvious that he
just had to quit."

"I realized," says Will, "that the goal of having a child
was most important. At that point, it wasn't a difficult decision to make."

Making Changes

Sallie and Will decided to join a weight-loss program as part of their effort to do all that they could to increase the likelihood of conception, because excess body fat can alter the balance of hormones that are crucial to reproduction. Their dietary goals were to cut back on fat intake and to eat more fruits and vegetables.

They started to eat out less. "We wanted to have more control over what we ate and how it was cooked," says Sallie, "and we had to cut back on our recreational expenses because of all we were spending on medical treatment."

Following through on their decision to eat healthier wasn't a problem, but sharing the kitchen was. "We had to learn to work together," says Will. "Each time we cooked, we had to decide who was kitchen boss for that meal."

For the most part, Will and Sallie agreed on the changes they wanted to make, so Sallie didn't have a lot of convincing to do. Having shared goals helped them both to stay committed.

There was, however, one goal that Sallie had but Will didn't share. She wanted to ask a therapist to help them sort through some problems that had existed in their relationship and were magnified by the stress that accompanies infertility. He didn't. "I wasn't very open to it," admits Will. "I didn't know what it was all about and what it would entail."

"I was at my wits' end," says Sallie, "but I didn't want to go to therapy alone. I didn't want to get more in tune with myself while my husband stayed in the same place. I felt our marriage depended on his coming with me, and I made that clear to him.

"There had been such a breakdown in our relationship that what I was suggesting was a solution, not a threat," she continues. "I didn't use it as a weapon. I simply said: 'If you have another idea of how to work on our relationship, I'm willing to listen. But if not, this is my idea. We need to try something.' " Not wanting to lose his marriage, Will finally agreed to try therapy.

Although Will felt defensive during the first few sessions, he eventually became convinced that the therapy could help. "It saved our marriage," he says in retrospect, "and I found it personally rewarding. The things I learned have helped me cope with problem situations in all areas of my life."

One of the things Will and Sallie came to realize was that their plan to start a family "wasn't happening," as Sallie puts it. "We decided we needed to get on with our lives; to do other things and not get stuck on this one thing," she says. The couple stopped medical treatment for infertility and thought about what they wanted their lives to be like.

Will was in a stressful job situation that he wanted to get out of. The couple didn't like living on Long Island because it was too crowded and built-up. They wanted to move to a New England state. So Sallie typed up Will's resumé and encouraged him to apply for a job that appeared to be a bit beyond his experience.

Was she pushing him so hard that it constituted nagging? "No," says Will. "The reason her pushing felt like encouragement rather than nagging was that I wanted to find a good job in a different place, too. It wasn't something Sallie wanted done that I had no interest in." The key was *shared goals*.

"It wasn't a negative thing," Sallie explains. "I wasn't

saying: 'You're fat. You're not perfect the way you are. Lose weight.' What I was saying was positive: 'I believe you're perfect for this job. I believe you can get the job you want.' "

This story has a happy ending. Will got the job in question, and the couple moved to Connecticut. They rented a home instead of buying one, which reduced their financial burden. Will was earning more money and wasn't coming home from work unhappy any more. Although Sallie had to give up her tenured teaching position in New York State, she made that sacrifice so that she and Will could begin to build the life they wanted.

Can Lifestyle Affect Fertility?

Within six months, Sallie discovered she was pregnant. In June 1993, she gave birth to a daughter. The couple now has three children. Does she believe that the lifestyle changes she and Will made to improve their health and reduce stress had anything to do with her three successful pregnancies after seven years of infertility?

"There's no question that as a couple we felt better," says Sallie. "It is certainly interesting that when we gave up on medical intervention, which is very stressful, and made some of these lifestyle changes, it happened.

"On the other hand," she continues, "I wouldn't want to give anyone the impression that if you have some serious medical problem, lifestyle changes will help you conceive. But in cases of unexplained fertility, like ours, living healthier may help. Following a nutritious diet, exercising, avoiding alcohol, not smoking, and reducing stress—it all seems to improve the chances of conception."

Improving the odds of conception isn't the only reason

for you and your partner to do what you can to enhance reproductive health. A healthy lifestyle also increases the odds of a healthy baby. Cigarette smoke, alcohol, and a diet high in sugar and low in nutrients can all be detrimental to a fetus.

Sallie's advice to couples trying to conceive: "Make sure you and your partner have the same goals. You need to know what your partner's priorities are, and he needs to know yours. That way, both of you can adjust your expectations and plans accordingly. In short, do your best to stay on the same team."

That advice is critical to success in virtually all areas of behavior change. Partners who make the *issue* the adversary, facing it as a team, have a much higher chance of achieving a happy ending than do partners who make adversaries of each other.

Impotence: A Common, Treatable Problem

Impotence—the inability to maintain an erection rigid enough to achieve mutually satisfying sexual intercourse— affects about one in 10 men and becomes more common with age. Researchers in Massachusetts found that 52 percent of men aged 40 to 70 had some degree of erectile impairment.

Many men and women mistakenly believe that impotence is chiefly a psychological problem. In reality, more than 75 percent of impotence cases are rooted in physical causes, including prostate problems, diabetes, vascular problems, hypertension, a low HDL ("good cholesterol") level, previous pelvic surgery, neurological disorders, hormone problems, injury, alcoholism, and drug abuse. In addition, certain medications can cause impotence. The remaining fourth of impotence cases do have psychological causes, including depression, stress, and performance anxiety.

Whatever the cause, about 95 percent of men with erectile dysfunction can be successfully treated. Unfortunately, only 10 percent of these men seek medical treatment. The most likely reason for men's reluctance to tell their doctors about impotence is embarrassment. Many men make a conscious or subconscious connection between manhood and erections. No wonder it's difficult for a man to call a doctor's office for an appointment, tell the receptionist the reason for his visit, then face a doctor who's going to ask him probing questions about this sensitive issue.

If your partner has erectile dysfunction, point out that it's a common problem, and state clearly that it's a problem you'll face together. Emphasize that impotence isn't a character flaw or a sign of reduced masculinity, it's a sign of an underlying health problem. That problem could be disease-based, mechanical, or a side effect of medication your man is taking for another condition.

Whether that problem turns out to be physical or psychological, chances are it's treatable. When impotence is caused by a disease such as diabetes or heart disease, getting medical help can save a man's life, not just his erection. Encourage your partner to talk about what he's feeling emotionally, and make sure that he knows you love him regardless. To reinforce the points you're making, or to get the conversation started, ask your partner to take the following impotence quiz.

HOW MUCH DO YOU KNOW ABOUT IMPOTENCE?
Take this test to see how much you know—and don't know—
about erectile dysfunction.

1. Impotence is defined as follows:
   a. Premature ejaculation
   b. Inability to achieve or sustain an erection
   c. Loss of manhood
2. Impotence can be caused by:
   a. Emotional conflict
   b. Injury
   c. Diabetes
   d. Side effects of prescription drugs
   e. All of the above
3. How many American men suffer from impotence?
   a. 10,000 to 20,000
   b. 1 to 5 million
   c. 10 to 20 million
4. Impotence can be a symptom of which of the following health problems:
   a. High blood pressure
   b. High cholesterol
   c. Heart disease
   d. All of the above
5. How many cigarettes does it take to have an effect on a man's ability to sustain an erection?
   a. 2
   b. 4
   c. 10
6. What percent of men between the ages of 40 and 70 are impotent to some degree?
   a. 16 percent
   b. 34 percent
   c. 52 percent

7. Impotence can be caused by medications you're taking.
   a. True
   b. False

8. Complete the following sentence: Impotence can be treated_____.
   a. rarely
   b. in most cases
   c. never

Answers:

1. B. Impotence is the inability to achieve or sustain an erection. It doesn't signify a loss of manhood, and it's not something you have to accept.

2. E. There are many causes for impotence. Fortunately, in almost all cases impotence can be treated successfully by a doctor.

3. C. Surprisingly, over 10 million men suffer from impotence in American alone. That's one in every 10 men.

4. D. Impotence is often a symptom of an underlying medical condition such as high blood pressure, high cholesterol, or heart disease.

5. A. Smoking as few as two cigarettes before having sex can affect a man's ability to achieve and sustain an erection.

6. C. Fifty-two percent of men in this age group suffer from impotence to some degree. That's one in every two men.

7. A. Impotence is often a side effect of medication or a symptom of an underlying physical condition.

8. B. Impotence can almost always be treated successfully by a doctor. Thanks to the variety of treatment options that are available today, most couples can enjoy intimate sexual contact once again.

Source: Pharmacia & Upjohn

How You Can Help Him Deal with Impotence

A simple act like offering to make a doctor's appointment for your partner will save him from having to give a stranger his name, then declare that he can't get an erection. Also offer to accompany him to the appointment for support. Many doctors acknowledge that a couple benefits more if both partners are involved in diagnosis and treatment of erectile dysfunction. However, if your man says that he'd prefer to go alone, don't argue.

Knowing what to expect from the visit will quell some of the anxiety your partner may be feeling. The first visit is designed to help the doctor determine the underlying medical condition or medication responsible for the impotence. It will likely start with a medical and sexual history. The doctor will want to know when and under what circumstances your partner experiences signs of impotence. The first visit will also include a physical examination, during which the doctor will check for abnormalities of the genitalia and prostate. Some basic laboratory tests—such as blood tests and urine analysis—will probably be ordered.

Viagra Frenzy

There are both medical and surgical treatment options for impotence. Certainly the most famous—or infamous— of the medical options is sildenafil citrate, otherwise known as Viagra. Approved by the Food and Drug Administration (FDA) in March 1998, Viagra got off to a rip-roaring start. In the first three months that it was available, 1.7 million prescriptions were written for 1 million patients.

But Viagra frenzy didn't stop there. Unusual stories began to creep into the news. An executive gave $1 million to a New York City hospital to buy Viagra for poor men. (Critics wondered if the money wouldn't have been better spent on life-saving medical treatments or potentially life-saving preventive screenings for those same men.) Samples of the drug disappeared at a meeting of an Israeli parliamentary science committee. Several brothels in Nevada reported that after Viagra arrived on the market, business increased by 10 to 20 percent. So many Canadians headed to Niagara Falls, New York, to buy the drug (which, at the time, wasn't available in Canada), that some observers suggested that the "Honeymoon Capital of the World" be given a new nickname: Viagra Falls.

However, it wasn't long before the world's enthusiasm for the new impotence defeating drug was dampened—however slightly—by the news of Viagra-related deaths. By early June 1998, 16 deaths had been reported by the FDA. Several of the deaths occurred in patients who suffered symptoms of heart attack after taking Viagra and were subsequently given nitroglycerin by emergency medical personnel. The medical care providers in these cases were either unaware that the two drugs are potentially lethal if combined, or they were unaware that the men they were treating had taken Viagra.

Viagra Cautions

Most of the other men who died after taking Viagra had histories of diabetes or heart disease, for which they were taking one or more medications. Some of those deaths might have occurred regardless of whether Viagra was taken. Others may have been related to the exertion of sexual intercourse, to which the men were unaccustomed, rather than directly to the drug itself.

These deaths make it clear that "borrowing" a pill that was prescribed for someone else would be foolhardy, indeed. Any man wishing to try Viagra must have a complete medical history and physical exam. In addition, nonexercisers with erectile dysfunction who would like to use Viagra should get into shape first. That will reduce the strain that sexual intercourse can put on the heart of a man who has been sedentary for a period of time.

Unlike other treatments for impotence, Viagra doesn't cause an erection directly. It works by enhancing the effects of nitric oxide, a chemical released in response to sexual stimulation that relaxes the smooth muscles in the penis. The relaxation of these muscles allows more blood to flow into the penis, which leads to an erection.

Viagra is taken an hour before intercourse, and should be used no more than once a day. Potential side effects include headache, flushing, indigestion, and altered color perception.

Psychotherapists and experts on sexuality have found that Viagra is causing emotional side effects, too. Although it might seem that the drug would improve a relationship affected by erectile dysfunction, it's not the magic bullet many people think it is. Viagra is relatively reliable and easy to use, but the little blue pill addresses only the physical barriers to sex, not the emotional barriers.

Many couples faced with impotence never fully explore what that problem means to them both as a couple and as individuals. With time, significant emotions get buried. When a drug comes along that makes intercourse possible in an unobtrusive and comfortable way, some couples find themselves staring at each other across an emotional chasm. Many are surprised to find that the resentment and pain caused by their damaged sex lives doesn't disappear with medication. Without professional help, it's hard for such couples to rebuild their relationships to the point where intercourse feels natural and desirable to both partners.

Beyond Viagra

Other treatment options for erectile dysfunction include erection-producing drugs that are injected into the penis or inserted in pellet form into the urethra before intercourse.

Vacuum erection devices can be used to simulate a natural erection mechanically. The penis is placed in a cylinder, and a handheld pump is used to suck blood into the erectile tissue of the penis. The erection is maintained by sliding, tight, elastic tubing around the base of the penis.

Penile prosthesis implantation is an option for some men. There are several varieties of penile implants. The simplest devices maintain stiffness, but don't increase the length or width of the penis. The most complex devices produce a more natural erection. Each variety carries pros and cons. Urologists can help patients choose the option that's right for them.

Prostate Problems

The prostate is a walnut-sized gland that sits under the bladder. The urethra, the tube that carries urine from the bladder to the penis and out of the body, runs through it. (Picture a minidoughnut with a straw inserted through the hole.) The prostate manufactures half of the fluid that makes up semen, which it secretes into the urethra prior to ejaculation.

The most common prostate problem is benign prostatic hyperplasia (BPH). Fifty percent of men over the age of 50 and 75 percent of those over the age of 70 suffer from BPH, commonly referred to as an enlarged prostate. When the prostate enlarges, it becomes more difficult for urine to pass through on its way out of the body. Symptoms of BPH include having to wait for the urine stream to get going, and a slower stream of urine once it comes. Because the bladder has to squeeze harder to eliminate urine, a man with an enlarged prostate may feel he has to urinate more often. At night this can be particularly annoying, making it difficult to get a good night's sleep.

BPH can be treated with medications designed to shrink the prostate gland or to improve the flow of urine by relaxing the tissues around the gland. If those fail, surgery may be required to reduce the size of the prostate.

 EIGHT REASONS YOUR MAN SHOULD SEE A DOCTOR
Early signs of prostate cancer are the same as the signs of many other disorders. If your partner notices any of the following symptoms, he should see a doctor:

1. Frequent urination (especially at night)
2. Inability to urinate
3. Trouble starting to urinate or trouble holding back urination
4. Pain during ejaculation
5. A weak or interrupted urine flow
6. Pain or a burning feeling during urination
7. Blood in the semen or in the urine
8. Frequent pain or stiffness in the lower back, hips, or upper thighs

The Infection Connection

Eventually, an enlarged prostate squeezes on the urethra so much that the bladder is strained, rendering it incapable of completely emptying itself. This makes the man feel that he has to go to the bathroom almost constantly. As time goes on, this situation can cause urine to back up into the kidneys, obstructing urine outflow from the kidneys and eventually leading to kidney damage. In addition, urine that remains in the bladder creates a breeding ground for bacteria that can cause an infection in the bladder or the prostate.

The symptoms of an acute prostate infection (called acute prostatitis) include sudden moderate to high fever; chills; frequent and difficult urination; urgent need to urinate; pain on urination; and pain in the lower back and in the area between the anus and the scrotum. Your partner should see a doctor immediately if he experiences any of those symptoms. Once an infection is confirmed, he'll be treated with antibiotics.

In some cases, a long-lasting or recurrent prostate infection or inflammation (called chronic prostatitis) follows an acute infection. Symptoms are milder than those of an acute infection. They include frequent need to urinate; urgent need to urinate; difficulty urinating; burning on urination; pain in the pelvis and in the genital area; and painful ejaculation. Medical treatment may involve long-term use of antibiotics, anti-inflammatory medication, and pain relievers.

Stanley has been dealing with BPH since 1985. He describes it as more of a nuisance than a real problem: "It means that I have to get up once or twice at night to urinate and also, of course, that I have to urinate more frequently during the day."

"The real problem," he continues, "arises when I get acute prostatitis, which happens about once a year. My already enlarged prostate gland balloons. When that happens, I have real difficulty urinating and feel the need to relieve myself every hour or even every 45 minutes. It has gotten so bad that I have found it almost impossible to urinate. In addition, I have a fever and chills, and in general feel pretty lousy."

A Team Effort

To avoid such unpleasant symptoms, Stanley does what he can to keep his prostate problems at bay. His wife Maggie, a retired registered nurse, helps in many ways. For example, she makes sure that he takes his Flomax, a medication prescribed to improve urinary flow.

Maggie does all the grocery shopping and she makes sure that there are very few items in the house that might irritate Stanley's prostate. "For example," he says, "I love tomato juice, but she never buys it because of its acidity. And I don't love it enough to go out and buy it myself!"

Maggie buys cranberry juice for Stanley because they've been told that it can help prevent the urinary tract infections that are common among men with BPH. She buys only decaffeinated coffee and rarely buys any caffeinated soft drinks. When cooking, Maggie uses spices moderately, and you won't find a salt or pepper shaker on the dinner table. The couple has stopped drinking hard liquor, although they still enjoy a glass of wine with dinner.

Another way Stanley tries to avoid prostatitis is by taking care to empty his bladder fully each time he uses the bathroom. He has noticed that not doing so can lead to an attack. "For example," he says, "we recently took a two-week car trip. We didn't want to make frequent pit stops, and we wanted to be quick when we did stop. That meant I had to 'hold it' more than usual and wasn't always able to completely empty my bladder. A week after we returned home, I had a major attack. Next time, we'll fly!"

What does Stanley hope the diet and habit changes he and Maggie have made will accomplish? "I believe the changes will enable me to reduce the frequency of acute prostatitis and, I hope, to avoid the need for a surgical remedy."

Indeed, many experts believe that pampering your prostate can make a difference. Another piece of good news for men with enlarged prostates is that BPH does not, as many people mistakenly believe, lead to prostate cancer.

A Common Cancer

Prostate cancer is the most common malignancy in men, accounting for about 30 percent of new cancer cases. From birth to death, American men have a one in five chance of developing prostate cancer. A slow-growing malignancy, it accounts for only 13 percent of cancer deaths in men, despite the frequency with which it occurs. By comparison, lung cancer accounts for just 15 percent of new cancer cases in men, but 32 percent of cancer deaths.

 RISK FACTORS FOR PROSTATE CANCER
According to the American Cancer Society, risk factors for prostate cancer include:

- **Age.** Prostate cancer is rare before the age of 50, but after 50 both incidence and mortality increase steadily.
- **Family history.** Having a father or brother with prostate cancer increases risk. According to one study, having a close female relative with breast cancer also increases risk.
- **Race.** African Americans develop the disease more frequently and have a worse prognosis than their white counterparts.
- **Heavy-metal exposure.** Prostate cancer is disproportionately high among workers with long-term exposure to high levels of cadmium (those who work in plants that make batteries, for example).
- **Diet.** Prostate cancer occurs more often in men whose diets are high in animal fat. Men whose diets are low in fruits, vegetables, and grains get more prostate cancer, too. Deficiencies of vitamin D and vitamin A have also been linked to increased risk.

Talk Openly about Reproductive Issues

Bringing reproductive issues into the open is the first step toward protecting reproductive health. Use the information in this chapter to start a discussion with your partner. Help him realize that his lifestyle choices can affect the health of one of his most prized organs and the systems that support it. Talk about your partner's family medical history and other risk factors that might affect his reproductive health. Discuss any problems that already exist, as well as your family-planning needs and goals. From there, you'll be able to select the changes listed in the beginning of this chapter that are most likely to benefit your partner and you. Then use information in the relevant chapters of this book to help your man make the changes he wants to make to protect his reproductive health.

7

HELP YOUR MAN KICK BUTTS

I want all hellions to quit puf ng that hell fume in God s clean air.

Carry Nation

Hell fume is an apt name for cigarette smoke. It causes more than 20 percent of all deaths from all diseases. Cigarettes kill more Americans than AIDS, alcohol abuse, car accidents, murders, suicides, drugs, and fires—combined. Tobacco use caused an estimated 3 million deaths worldwide in 1990. By 2020, that number is expected nearly to triple to 8.4 million people a year.

What can you do to prevent your partner from becoming a smoking statistic? Why is it so hard for smokers to quit? Exactly how does your partner's smoking affect his health—and his family's? We'll answer those questions—and more—in this chapter.

Of the more than 4,000 chemicals cigarette smoke contains, 43 are known to promote cancer. Every time a smoker lights up, he exposes the delicate tissues of the mouth, throat, voice box, bronchi (air tubes in the lungs), and the lungs themselves to those cancer-causing chemicals. In addition, smoke damages the alveoli (tiny air sacs in the lungs where carbon dioxide is exchanged for oxygen). Eventually, these tubes and/or sacs can become so damaged that they're unable to carry adequate levels of oxygen to the vital organs. The result is death from emphysema or chronic bronchitis.

Cigarette smoke is the cause of about 25 percent of deaths from coronary artery disease. The nicotine in cigarettes increases blood pressure and heart rate temporarily, causing the heart to work harder. In addition, the carbon monoxide in cigarettes binds with hemoglobin, displacing oxygen and depriving the heart of that vital element. Smoking causes platelets (colorless blood cells whose job it is to plug holes in injured blood vessels) to clump together, thus contributing to atherosclerosis (clogging of the arteries), which causes heart attacks and strokes. The bottom line is that smoking a pack of cigarettes a day puts as much strain on the heart as does gaining 80 to 90 pounds.

MORE REASONS TO BE SMOKE FREE

Although lung cancer, heart disease, emphysema, and bronchitis are the most common diseases people get from smoking, they aren't the only ones. Here are some additional maladies that are caused or aggravated by cigarette smoke:

- Smoking is a major cause of cancer of the mouth, larynx, esophagus, stomach, kidney, bladder, pancreas, uterus, and cervix.
- Smokers are more likely than nonsmokers to have back problems such as pain, sciatica, and degenerative disease of the spine. (Chronic tobacco use weakens the bones.)
- Smoking constricts blood vessels in the penis (and throughout the body), substantially increasing the risk of erectile dysfunction.
- Smoking reduces sperm count and motility.

- Smoking accelerates the process of rheumatoid arthritis, a chronic inflammation and degeneration of joints.
- Smoking causes cosmetic damage, such as wrinkles, gray hair, and hair loss.

What Factors Help a Smoker Quit?

That's a question to which there are as many answers as there are smokers. Because cigarette smoke is so highly addictive (about five times more addictive than cocaine), it takes more to break the smoking habit than it does, say, to start drinking orange juice with your breakfast every morning. Although there are many things a woman can do to help her man kick the habit, he has to have a strong desire to beat his addiction, or it's unlikely that he'll do so.

Dennis Diemond was only 21 when he was diagnosed with leukemia. Once he was in remission, he was scheduled to fly from his home in a suburb of Boston to Seattle for a bone-marrow transplant. The night before he left, he asked one of the nurses who had cared for him in the hospital to marry him. She flew with him to Seattle and helped care for him through some difficult complications that resulted from the transplant. Two years later, when Dennis was fully recovered, he and Grace were married.

"It was a very difficult time for both of us," says Grace Diemond. "But if he hadn't gotten sick, we'd never have met." Dennis quit smoking cigarettes in 1981, right before his bone-marrow transplant. Around 1988, he started to smoke again, but not around Grace.

"If I got in the truck and smelled smoke," says Grace, "I'd call him on it. He'd say that a friend had been smoking in the truck. His siblings used to tell me that he was smoking when I wasn't around. Finally, I just said to him: 'You're not fooling me, and you're not hurting me because you're not smoking around me. But you're hurting yourself.' We had our battles about it."

Being a nurse, Grace was well equipped to describe the dangers of smoking. "I would say to him: 'It's your choice; you're an adult. But this is what could happen if you choose to continue smoking.' "

She maintained her hands-off approach, understanding that quitting was something he would do himself when the time was right. That time came when Dennis's father, also a smoker, was diagnosed with emphysema and then lung cancer. "Dennis saw his father, a robust six-foot man, in the hospital struggling for breath. He said to me: 'If smoking can do this to my Dad, it can do the same to me.' " In 1995, Dennis quit smoking cold turkey and hasn't had a cigarette since.

Surprisingly, the trauma of seeing someone you love with a smoking-related illness—or even having one yourself—doesn't always do the trick. In fact, only about 50 percent of smokers who have a heart attack quit smoking, despite the fact that smoking significantly increases heart-attack risk.

Lisa and David Mandozzi were both smokers before their first child was born. "I had tried to quit while I was pregnant," she says, "but all I managed to do was to cut back. I knew smoking was bad for the baby and for me, but it all seemed so abstract. It wasn't until I held him in my arms that I fully understood that there had been a little person growing inside me."

QUIT FOR THE KIDS

Parents who smoke need only look across their kitchen table to be reminded of the most compelling reason to quit smoking—

their children's health. Nevertheless, 43 percent of American children live in a household with someone who smokes tobacco. Here's how passive smoking threatens children's health:

- An infant who is exposed to cigarette smoke during gestation or after birth is at increased risk of sudden infant death syndrome (SIDS).
- More young people are killed by parental smoking than by all other unintentional injuries combined.
- Among infants to 18 months of age, secondhand smoke is associated with as many as 300,000 cases of bronchitis and pneumonia each year.
- Children raised in a smoking environment have higher rates of asthma, more respiratory problems, and more ear infections than those raised in a nonsmoking environment.
- Passive smoking reduces a child's HDL cholesterol level by about 10 percent. (HDL is the good cholesterol that helps to reduce damaging LDL cholesterol in the blood, thus protecting the heart.)
- If both parents smoke, a teenager is more than twice as likely to smoke than a young person whose parents are both nonsmokers. If one parent smokes, the likelihood that a teenager will smoke also is increased.

A Tale of Two Quitters

As soon as the baby arrived, Lisa quit smoking. "The baby gave me the power to quit," she explains. David, however, still wasn't ready. Like virtually all adult smokers, he had started to smoke at a young age, in his case at 13. Getting hooked young makes quitting that much harder.

David was well aware that he needed to give up cigarettes both to support his wife who was working so hard to stay smoke-free, and to protect the health of their son. In addition, he had his own health to worry about: David's older brother died of a massive heart attack at the age of 32.

How did Lisa help David give up smoking? "I knew that he knew he had to quit," she says. "I just tried to support him. When he did decide to quit, it was easier for him because I wasn't smoking." Seven months after Michael was born, David went to a hypnotist. After one visit, he began to cut back and eventually he quit completely.

Meanwhile, Lisa wasn't having an easy time. "Quitting smoking was the hardest thing I've ever had to do," she says. "It was a nasty, nasty year, but when it was over, I felt strong for having done it."

How did she and David cope with the symptoms they experienced? Lisa started to exercise more, and eventually began teaching aerobics. Now she's the director of fitness at a YMCA in Massachusetts. David didn't follow suit until two years after Michael was born. "When he quit," says Lisa, "he was so uptight and tense that I finally told him to join a club and work out before coming home at night.

"Now," she says with a laugh, "it's like: 'Will you please come home from the gym?' Exercising really helps him decompress at the end of the day. It helps him make the transition from work to home."

One of the best things a would-be quitter can do is to avoid situations in which he or she would normally light up. For example, one of Lisa's smoking habits was to light up while talking on the phone to friends. "I actually lost touch with some friends because I couldn't stay on the phone for more than three minutes without craving a cigarette."

Other smokers like to light up when they're driving, after dinner, or when socializing in a bar or restaurant. "You have to allow for some change in your routine," says Lisa. "If your partner needs to avoid certain situations, avoid them with him."

 STARTLING STATISTICS

Take a look at these smoking statistics and share them with your partner. About half a million Americans die every year of smoking-related diseases and accidents. Researchers in North Carolina found that, although smokers are aware that they're putting their health in jeopardy, they underestimate the extent to which lighting up increases their risk of disease and death—and yours.

- Number of people alive today who will eventually be killed by tobacco: half a billion.
- Number of American smokers who die of diseases caused by smoking each year: 419,000.
- Number of American nonsmokers who die of diseases caused by second-hand smoke each year: 53,000.
- Number of deaths each year in the U.S. caused by fires that were started by cigarettes: 25,000.
- Number of children poisoned (nonfatally) by eating cigarette butts in 1995: 8,000.
- Number of minutes every cigarette smoked shaves off the smoker's life: 12.
- Percentage of American men who smoke: 28.
- Percentage of African-American men who smoke: 34.
- Number of Americans who try to quit smoking each year: 17 million.
- Number who succeed: 1.2 million.
- Number of American adolescents who smoke cigarettes: 3 million.
- Number of American adolescents each day who try their first cigarette: 3,000.

An Addiction Like Any Other

Given that smoking drastically increases risk of chronic illness, and that one in four smokers will die early because of the habit, why on earth do people smoke? There are physiological and psychological reasons people become addicted to cigarettes. Understanding these reasons will improve your ability to provide useful support and encouragement to a smoker who's trying to quit.

First, let's be clear: nicotine is a drug, and a highly addictive one at that. As one former tobacco-company researcher has said: "It's just like putting a needle in your arm and pushing something in."

Recently released internal documents from tobacco companies revealed that cigarette makers have known for decades that nicotine is addictive, and that the companies were acutally manipulating the nicotine level in cigarettes to make them more addictive.

How does nicotine affect the brain and cause people to get hooked? Researchers at New York's Columbia-Presbyterian Medical Center found that it stimulates the release of the brain's neurotransmitters—chemicals that carry messages from one nerve ending to another. The result is heightened alertness, an increased sense of pleasure, and improved short-term memory. One of the study's investigators explained the effect of nicotine on the brain this way: "It's just like turning up the volume on a radio."

Research strongly suggests that dopamine, a neurotransmitter associated with feelings of pleasure and elation, is the "master molecule of addiction." Nicotine, as well as drugs such as cocaine, heroin, amphetamines, and alcohol, stimulates dopamine-producing cells to pump out more of the chemical. The result is that the person ingesting these substances feels good. In effect, the brain rewards their behavior.

While nicotine pumps up the production of dopamine, scientists theorize that another, as-yet unidentified chemical in cigarette smoke increases the length of time dopamine remains in circulation. It does this by blocking the action of MAO-B, an enzyme that would normally destroy dopamine.

This research points up the fact that, contrary to what many Americans believe, cigarette smoking isn't simply a weakness of character; it's a disorder of the brain that has its roots in chemical reactions, just like other mental disorders. Many researchers believe that some people are genetically predisposed to addiction because of an inherited brain abnormality that limits the production of dopamine.

In fact, there are links between nicotine addiction and other mental health problems. Several studies have found that smokers are more likely than nonsmokers to suffer from depression, anxiety disorder, eating disorders, and attention deficit hyperactivity disorder (ADHD). Nicotine's boosting effect on neurotransmitters such as dopamine, serotonin, and norepinephrin may help reduce a person's psychiatric symptoms, making it extremely hard for them to give up cigarettes.

People who use nicotine are more likely than those who don't to use other mood-altering drugs as well. In fact, the best way to deal with the nation's *illicit* drug problem would be to sharply reduce the use of *licit* drugs—primarily alcohol and tobacco—by children and teenagers.

Dealing with Depression

If your partner shows symptoms that might indicate depression (see "Symptoms of Depression," page 206) or anxiety, he should address that health concern before trying to quit smoking. Although little talked about, depression is one of the most common medical illnesses, affecting more than 17 million Americans each year. Only about one-third of depressed people seek treatment. That's unfortunate, because 80 to 90 percent of them could be helped with a combination of medication and therapy.

How can you help? If you think your partner might be depressed, don't offer simplistic reassurances like: "Things will all work out for the best." Instead, listen attentively and understand that no matter how unrealistic his concerns may seem to you, they're real to him. Emphasize that depression is a common and highly treatable illness. Offer to go along to a doctor's appointment with your partner if you think it would make the visit easier for him.

 SYMPTOMS OF DEPRESSION

According to the National Institutes of Mental Health, common symptoms of severe depression include:

- Marked changes in sleep pattern (sleeping less or more than usual)
- Decreased appetite and weight loss or, conversely, increased appetite and weight gain
- Persistent sad, anxious, or "empty" moods
- Feelings of hopelessness and pessimism
- Feelings of guilt, worthlessness, and helplessness
- Fatigue or decreased energy
- Difficulty concentrating
- Thoughts or talk of death or suicide; suicide threats or attempts

Other, more subtle, symptoms of depression include:

- Changes in social behavior, such as going out less, avoiding friends, and talking less with family members at home
- Frequent overreaction—for example: taking offense when none was intended; perceiving minor difficulties as major road blocks
- Forgetfulness—such as having to check the time of an appointment repeatedly or forgetting family plans
- Declining appearance—a depressed person may start paying less attention to personal grooming, and dressing less neatly
- Chronic indecision—ongoing difficulty with things like choosing a meal from a menu or deciding on a gift for a friend's birthday
- Mysterious pains—these may include stomachaches, muscle aches, and joint pain that don't respond to treatment

Anxiety and Smoking

Anxiety is as common as depression. Symptoms include a feeling of always being keyed up and extra-alert; shortness of breath; racing heart; and restlessness. These reactions would be considered normal in certain situations, such as starting a new job or moving. However, if a person feels anxiety that's out of proportion with what's happening in his life or is interfering with his relationships or his ability to work, he should seek help from a doctor.

People with anxiety may smoke because it helps them feel calmer. However, in addition to being dangerous, smoking is just a temporary fix. What's needed is a long-term solution for anxiety. In most cases, as with depression, that means a combination of psychotherapy and medication.

You can help a partner who has heightened anxiety in many ways. As with other areas of behavior change, set a good example yourself. For example, allow yourself five extra minutes to get where you're going, whether it's to work or to a movie. Encourage him to develop the same habit. It will reduce your risk of being late, a possibility that increases anxiety for most of us. Likewise, it's a good idea to allow a little more time to complete a given task than you think it will take. For example, if your partner estimates that it will take him half a day to complete this year's tax return, suggest that he set aside a full day (or two half days) at least a week before April 15. That way he'll have time to research any unexpected questions that come up.

Task overload makes many people anxious. Suggest to your mate that you and he reduce the number of things you each try to accomplish in a day. Also make a concerted effort to avoid doing more than one thing at a time.

When anxiety does creep in, remind your man to ask himself this question: "What's the worst thing that could happen?" Usually, the answer is something quite unterrifying. In the case of being late for work, for example, it might be: "I'll have to stay a few minutes later than usual to make up the time."

Seeking treatment for depression or anxiety, and learning to manage the thoughts and beliefs that help to create those states of mind, will help a smoker reduce his "need" for cigarettes.

Help for Smokers Who Want to Quit

According to the Centers for Disease Control and Prevention, of the more than 15 million American adults who try to quit smoking each year, only about 8 percent succeed at any one time. That's a pretty discouraging statistic; however, overall, about 40 percent of all people who have ever smoked have managed to quit, although it takes most smokers a number of attempts before they become ex-smokers permanently.

How can you help ensure that your man quits smoking successfully? The key, experts agree, is to get help from several sources. A doctor can prescribe medication that will help your partner break his addiction. A support group will teach him the skills he needs to remain smoke free. There are short-term quitting courses given by chapters of the American Cancer Society and the American Lung Association as well as by many local hospitals, which many would-be quitters find very helpful. Friends and family can assist by inviting your man on smoke-free outings (to museums, movies, or plays, for example) instead of gathering at a restaurant or bar.

Here's a rundown of some of the medications that can be used to reduce the withdrawal symptoms that smokers experience when they give up cigarettes. These aids help to ease the quitter through the difficult first weeks of being smoke-free.

• *Nicotine gum.* Nicotine-containing chewing gum allows smokers to give up cigarettes without putting an abrupt stop to their intake of nicotine, a move that could cause difficult withdrawal symptoms. Quitters chew the gum throughout the day as needed, gradually reducing the frequency of use until the gum is no longer needed. Nicotine gum is available over the counter. One advantage that nicotine gum has over a nicotine patch is that a patch sometimes irritates the skin to which it's applied. Some people like the way they can self-dose with gum, popping a piece in their mouths when the urge to smoke strikes.

A note of caution: users of nicotine gum should be certain to follow directions. That means chewing a full dose for two to three months, a lower dose for two to three months more, then switching to sugarless gum or no gum at all. It's important to note that nicotine gum shouldn't be considered a permanent replacement for cigarettes. Its continued use for one year or more has been shown to increase risk of diabetes and heart disease.

• *Nicotine patch.* Nicotine patches are also available over the counter. Many people find them more convenient than gum because, in most cases, users apply a patch once every 24 hours and then can forget about it—no need to carry a pack of gum around or to chew gum at work. In one study, 27 percent of smokers who used nicotine patches were still not smoking six months later. Only 13 percent of smokers who were given placebo patches continued to abstain from smoking after six months.

A note of caution: be sure to dispose of used patches where young children can't get at them, and to instruct children that the patches contain medicine and should not be played with or sucked on. U.S. poison-control centers have reported incidents in which children chewed or bit patches or placed them on their skin, resulting in symptoms such as nausea, vomiting, diarrhea, abdominal pain, dizziness, weakness, and rash.

• *Nicotine nasal spray.* Nasal sprays get nicotine into the bloodstream faster than the patch or gum. They're available by prescription only.

• *Bupropion HCI.* This drug is packaged under the brand name Zyban as a smoking-cessation aid, and under the brand name Wellbutrin as an antidepressant. Why does the same drug work for both nicotine addiction and depression? No one knows for certain, but scientists speculate that the drug helps people with both diseases by inhibiting the reabsorption into the body of mood-elevating neuro-transmitters such as dopamine. With more dopamine in circulation, smokers may suffer less when they give up cigarettes, which makes it easier to quit.

In a study of more than 600 smokers, 44 percent of those who received Zyban kicked the habit versus 19 percent of patients who didn't receive the drug. In addition, average weight gain among those taking Zyban was 3.3 pounds, compared to 6.4 pounds among those not taking it.

 HOW AN EX-SMOKER'S BODY THANKS HIM
If you hear the common argument: "It's too late; the damage is done" from your partner, share with him this list of improvements that occur when a smoker quits:

- Within 24 hours of quitting, the level of carbon monoxide and nicotine in a smoker's system decreases rapidly. Smoking's negative effects on bronchitis will begin to be reversed, and those with emphysema will find it easier to breath. Although emphysema isn't reversible, quitting smoking slows the progress of the disease.
- Within a few days of quitting, an ex-smoker's senses of taste and smell start to improve; he may breathe easier and notice improvement in his stamina. Smoker's cough will begin to abate.
- Within two years of quitting, a former smoker's risk of heart attack is reduced by about 24 percent; within five years, his risk is reduced by 50 to 70 percent; and within 10 to 14 years, his risk level is almost equal with someone who never smoked.
- Quitting smoking immediately decreases the chance of esophageal or pancreatic cancer.
- Within seven years, risk of bladder cancer drops to that of a nonsmoker.
- After 10 to 15 years, an ex-smoker's risk of getting cancer of the lung, larynx, or mouth is close to that of a lifetime nonsmoker's.

How to Handle Nicotine Withdrawal

It's a fact of life—quitting an addictive chemical leads to withdrawal symptoms. Although there's no way to avoid these symptoms, there are things one can do to minimize their effects. The following list is reprinted courtesy of the Washington State branch of Doctors Ought to Care.

Symptom: Irritability

Cause: Heavy smokers are more likely to report this symptom. The irritability people experience after quitting is caused by the body's craving for nicotine.

Solution: Try nicotine chewing gum, a nicotine patch, relaxing exercise, a warm shower, or a brisk walk. Irritability associated with quitting will lessen over time. (Average duration is two to four weeks.)

Symptom: Fatigue

Cause: Nicotine is a stimulant, so it's not surprising that quitting smoking causes fatigue. Heavy smokers are more likely to feel tired after quitting. Fatigue is likely to occur in the afternoon from 2 P.M. to 4 P.M.

Solution: Try nicotine gum or a nicotine patch, take naps or a brisk walk.

Symptom: Insomnia

Cause: Nicotine affects brain wave functioning and may influence sleep patterns. It's not uncommon in the first few days after quitting for the ex-smoker to wake up frequently during the night. Dreaming about smoking is also common. Coughing after quitting also may contribute to wakefulness.

Solution: Avoid caffeine after 6 P.M. and try relaxation techniques. This symptom rarely lasts longer than a week after quitting.

Symptom: Depression

Cause: It's not uncommon to feel a little depressed after quitting tobacco. Some say that quitting smoking is like losing a close friend. Bouts of crying are not uncommon.

Solution: Understand that the feelings are normal and will pass. Talk to a friend, write a letter to yourself, or volunteer at a hospital, an animal shelter, or another place where you can help others.

Symptom: Tightness in the chest

Cause: It's not uncommon to experience a tightness in the chest after quitting. Chest tightness is probably due to the tension created by the body's need for nicotine. Chest tightness occurs more often in those who report ex-smoker's cough, which may mean that the chest muscles are sore from coughing.

Solution: Try relaxation techniques, especially deep breathing. Nicotine gum or the patch may help. This symptom passes within a few days after quitting.

Symptom: Stomach pains, constipation, gas

Cause: Intestinal movement may decrease for a brief

period when a smoker lowers his or her tobacco use.

Solution: Eat lots of roughage, like raw fruits and vegetables and whole-grain breads and cereals. Drink
six to eight glasses of water each day. Exercise.

Symptom: Hunger

Cause: The craving for a cigarette is often confused with
hunger pangs. As a result, many people find
themselves eating more after quitting. Heavy
tobacco users experience feelings of hunger
more often after quitting than light users.

Solution: Try nicotine gum, a nicotine patch, low calorie snacks, or beverages. This symptom is
usually most intense in the first week after
quitting and may persist for several weeks.

Symptom: Coughing; dry throat

Cause: Ex-smoker's cough is the body's way of getting rid of the extra mucus that has blocked
airways. Dry throat is caused by the fact that
the body is no longer producing a lot of
mucus to protect the airways from the toxins.

Solution: Try drinking cold water, fruit juice, or tea. Chew
gum or suck on cough drops or hard candy.

Symptom: Dizziness

Cause: The occasional dizziness that some ex-smokers experience is caused by the extra oxygen
that the body is getting.

Solution: Take extra caution in the things that you do.
Change positions slowly. This symptom rarely
lasts longer than a day or two after quitting.

Symptom: Lack of concentration

Cause: Nicotine affects brain-wave functioning. Recent studies indicate that concentration and problem-solving ability are enhanced in smokers for a short period (20 to 30 minutes) following administration of nicotine. Changing a habit as ingrained as smoking takes effort and contributes to problems in concentration. The tobacco user's body needs time to adjust to a routine of not having constant stimulation from nicotine.

Solution: Plan your workload to account for your temporary lack of concentration. Avoid additional stress during the first few weeks. Most former tobacco users say that concentration isn't a problem after a few weeks of being tobacco-free.

A Band-Aid for Smokers

If the time isn't right for your partner to quit smoking, encourage him to take up or continue to exercise. Swedish researchers found that smokers who participated in vigorous physical activity (running, tennis, swimming, or similar activities for at least two hours per week) had a 40-percent lower risk of dying of a heart attack or stroke than smokers who were sedentary. However, bear in mind that smokers who exercise are still four times as likely to die as nonsmokers who exercise.

If your partner does decide to quit, realize that quitting smoking may well make for, as Lisa Mandozzi put it, "a nasty, nasty year." Lisa advises other women who want to help their mates quit smoking to be as understanding as

INTERNET RESOURCES

• **Nicotine Anonymous:** http://nicotine-anonymous.org **or:** http://www.nicotine-anonymous.org. (The sites are identical). This is the official site of the 12-step program for those who wish to quit smoking. It lists the 12 steps to smoking cessation (adapted from the 12-step list developed by Alcoholics Anonymous), explains the program, and gives tips for would-be quitters. The site also includes a directory of meetings in the U.S. (by state and city), and a directory of international meetings.

• **American Lung Association:** http://www.lungusa.org. To access the ALA's online smoking-cessation clinic, click on "participate", then "programs", then "Freedom From Smoking", and finally, "Freedom From Smoking on-line". Freedom From Smoking is an individualized program that takes into account such personal factors as why you smoke, when you smoke and with whom you smoke. The program consists of seven online clinics, for which there is a fee of $45 "as a gesture of commitment." Participants quit smoking at session three. The remaining sessions are dedicated to offering support and to helping participants adapt to a nonsmoking lifestyle. A work-book version of the program is also available. Call 1–800–LUNG–USA for more information.

• **Quit Smoking Today!:** http://home1.gte.net/kclement/qstoday/index.htm. This site offers an extensive list of links to medical societies, government agencies and other organizations related to smoking cessation.

• **Blair's Quitting Smoking Resources:** http://www.chriscor.com/linkstoa.htm. An extensive list of useful Internet sites put together by a Canadian who says that the information she gathered on the Internet helped her to quit smoking. The site also includes a chat room, a bulletin board and a quitting smoking bookstore.

possible about how difficult it is to quit. "Keep encouraging him even if he has a relapse," she says. "For some people, that's part of the quitting process." Experts agree that every attempt at quitting teaches a smoker more about what it will take to quit successfully. If your partner has a relapse, emphasize that a relapse isn't a failure; it's a learning step. Don't give up on your man. Remain supportive and show that you believe he'll eventually become smoke-free.

TEN WAYS TO SUPPORT AN EX-SMOKER
In addition to encouraging your man to consult his doctor about quitting and to find a support group or quitter's course with which he's comfortable, use the following 10 techniques to support a would-be ex-smoker:

1. Ask your partner how you can help. Often, the smoker himself knows how you can assist him best. Maybe he needs someone he can talk to about how he feels physically and mentally. Perhaps he would rather that you distract him by planning fun activities or being his workout partner. If he associates coffee with smoking, you may have to give up your morning cup for a while.

2. Don't underestimate the power of praise. If your man is a newly minted ex-smoker, tell him how fresh his breath smells, and that he himself smells good, too. If you've noticed an increase in his stamina, make sure he knows about it. Tell him that you're proud that he got through another day without lighting up.

3. Help your man avoid temptation. Don't meet friends at bars or at restaurants without no-smoking sections. Instead, suggest a museum, a sporting event, or a movie. If your man is used to lighting up whenever he talks on the phone, ask friends not to call for a month unless they have a specific purpose that can be handled quickly. If it's driving that sparks your partner's nicotine craving, don't plan any long car trips for a month or two.

4. Don't linger at the table after a meal at home. Instead, focus on what you'll do after dinner. "After we eat, let's climb into bed and read," or "let's go out for a walk," or "let's get on the Internet and plan our next vacation."

5. Help your ex-smoker develop new habits or interests to replace smoking. It's important for those giving up cigarettes to have something to turn their attention to when a craving hits. Taking up exercise is the best solution. Not only does it keep a former smoker's mind off cigarettes while he's doing it, but it will help relieve some of the possible symptoms of quitting, such as depression, irritability, fatigue, weight gain, and constipation. If he's already exercising, encourage him to take up a new hobby that will keep his hands busy. For example, he might take up drawing, woodworking, car repair, photography, or the guitar.

6. Help your partner choose a "quit date." Pick a target date that doesn't fall during a holiday or at the time of an important family party like a reunion or a wedding. Big occasions make smoking a big temptation. The first day is critical. Researchers in North Carolina found that of 207 pack-a-day smokers, those who refrained from smoking on day one were 10 times more likely to remain smoke-free after six months than those who sneaked a cigarette on their quit date.

7. Find an ex-smoker's support group that he'll feel comfortable in. Check your local Yellow Pages, ask your doctor, or call your local hospital. The Internet is an option for those who can't see themselves attending a meeting in person. (See "Internet Resources" on page 212.)

8. Be tolerant. Many smokers get cranky, depressed, or anxious after they quit. Put up with these moods as best you can—they will pass.

9. Tell your partner not to worry about weight gain. The average male smoker who quits gains just nine pounds, an amount that can easily be lost once your partner is established as a nonsmoker. If he's concerned about weight gain, point out that a little excess weight is far less dangerous to his health than smoking cigarettes. In fact, the average person would have to gain 80 to 90 pounds to place the same amount of strain on his heart that a pack-a-day habit does. Point out that walking an extra mile every day will burn 100 calories—enough to help offset weight gain. Offer to walk with him.

10. Help your partner pick a reward. Plan something for your man to look forward to at the end of his first smoke-free year. It might be a dream vacation for the two of you, a new mountain bike, a computer, a camera, or some other item he's been wanting.

8

DE-EMPHASIZE ALCOHOL

Nothing in excess.
Inscribed on the oracle
at the Temple of Apollo, Delphi

For many people, that simple advice isn't so simple to follow. In American culture, alcohol has become a tonic for grief and stress, as well as an integral part of celebrations such as weddings, family reunions, and job promotions. In addition, alcohol acts as a lubricant in social situations, making parties livelier and conversations more revealing. For some people, alcohol can even become an integral part of work.

"Drinking and sales go hand in hand," says Rich Canady, a 39-year-old father of three. "Not only is alcohol readily available at business lunches and dinners, but the company picks up the tab. Some clients want you to have a drink with them, and it's harder to connect with them if you don't. In fact, after I had given up alcohol, one customer actually got upset because I ordered a soda at lunch."

How One Drink Becomes Five

Liquor was also part of Rich's home life. "When I came through the door in the evening, I needed a drink," he says, "what with the stress of the work day plus the kids jumping on me. One drink would turn into four or five, and I'd find myself waking up on a Tuesday with hangover. I made Tylenol rich, taking two or three tablets a day. I fell into that trap for about eight years. It got so bad that I felt like my liver was shivering."

Rich's wife, Val, would occasionally question his level of drinking and ask when he was planning to cut back. She told Rich that she was concerned about the effects the alcohol was having on his physical and mental health. Rich admits that his drinking was causing problems in the family. "I was lashing out at the kids, and pushing Val away from me emotionally," he says.

Today, Rich doesn't drink a drop of alcohol. He eats a low-fat diet rich in fruits and vegetables, and exercises nearly every day. Two events left Rich determined to make those lifestyle changes. The first occurred in 1996, when he had a routine physical examination. "I weighed in at over 350 pounds," he says. "I was deemed 'obese.' I had never thought of myself that way before, even though I couldn't walk two blocks without stopping for breath. I wondered: 'How did I let myself get to this point?' I felt so bad that I wanted to cry."

Then, on a Sunday morning in February 1997, Rich woke up with a sharp tugging pain on the left side of his abdomen, and noticed blood in his stool. Nevertheless, he spent the afternoon drinking rum and cokes while watching a basketball game on television. At one point, he realized how odd it was that he kept drinking even though he didn't feel well. On Monday morning, Rich decided to see a doctor.

The diagnosis was diverticulitis, an infection in the large intestine (colon) that occurs when diverticula (small, abnormal pouches that bulge outward from the wall of the colon at a point of weakness) become inflamed or rupture. Most often, the disease can be treated with antibiotics, but some cases require surgery.

"Being sick was a significant emotional event for me," says Rich. "I never felt so much pain. When I looked up diverticulitis in a medical book and read that it could lead to peritonitis, which can be fatal, I was really shaken."

Rich was told not to drink alcohol while taking the antibiotic his doctor prescribed. "That was the first week I went without liquor," he says. "One day that week I said to myself: 'Let me just go for a walk.' " Soon, Rich was working out at a gym on a regular basis. There he became friendly with a man who invited him to church. Rich and his family now attend that church every Sunday. "Religion has really helped," says Rich. "Jesus inspires me to be kinder and more giving. I just keep praying for his help."

Val helps Rich, too. She puts out a breakfast of fresh fruit every morning and keeps the kitchen stocked with low-fat, healthy snacks and plenty of nonalcoholic beverages. "Just to have her setting me up in my daily routine helps a lot," says Rich.

She gives Rich free rein to spend time at the gym, taking care of the children and keeping the household clean and organized. But most of all, says Rich, Val helps by encouraging him. "She tells me she's proud of me, and that means a lot."

"I try to help him along with positive encouragement," says Val, "and he has a very nice network of family and friends who encourage him and praise him."

A great way for a woman to help her man cut back on drinking is to help him avoid situations that make him want to drink. It's important to replace old habits that went hand in hand with drinking with new habits that don't. "When you give up something, you have to replace it," says Val. "Rich has replaced drinking with exercise, church, and family activities."

 INTERNET RESOURCES
For more information on alcohol and alcoholism, check these Web sites:

• **Another Empty Bottle:** http://www.alcoholismhelp.com/help/. This site is intended for the friends and family of alcoholics. It features links, a discussion area, a page for children, and a list of resources for problems that often accompany alcoholism, such as depression and domestic violence.

• **National Council on Alcoholism and Drug Dependence:** http://www.ncadd.org/. A good source of facts about alcoholism and alcohol-related health information. This site also includes a message board, a resource and referral guide, and information for parents on how to talk to children about alcohol.

• **Al-Anon and Alateen:** http://www.al-anon.org/. This is the official U.S. Web site for two organizations: Al-Anon (for adult family and friends of alcoholics), and Alateen (for teenage children of alcoholics). It includes information about 12-step programs and offers related books for purchase on line. Also available here is a directory of groups in Canada and the U.S.

• **Alcoholics Anonymous:** http://www.alcoholics-anonymous.org/. AA is a society of more than 2 million recovered alcoholics. This Web site offers basic information about who might benefit from this 12-step program, and how the program works.

Seeking Support

Rich was fortunate to be able to stop drinking on his own—without simply replacing one intoxicating drug with another, such as marijuana or cocaine. However, many people need help from Alcoholics Anonymous or from an employee assistance program.

A woman can do many things to encourage her mate to become involved in such a program. Initially, she can find out the name and phone number of a local contact person and the times and locations of meetings. Later, she can go to meetings with her partner and/or go independently to meetings of alcoholic codependents. (A codependent is a person who isn't herself addicted, but who is thoroughly involved in—and thus curiously supportive of—her partner's addiction.)

Last but not least, a woman who would like her partner to drink less alcohol needs to drink less herself. "I've cut back significantly," says Val. Although she still has a glass of wine on an occasional Saturday night, more often she opts for hot chocolate or joins Rich in a glass of seltzer water or grapefruit juice. When the couple hosts a party, which they often do, they no longer supply any alcoholic beverages. "Now Rich just tells everyone: 'If you want something to drink, you'll have to bring it yourselves,'" says Val. "No one is offended. Everyone is proud of what Rich has accomplished."

 THREE SIGNS OF A DRINKING PROBLEM
If you think your partner may be abusing alcohol, watch for these three changes that typically signal a drinking problem:

1. Changes in mood and behavior. A person who has always been attentive may become distracted and have difficulty carrying on a group conversation. He may interject unrelated ideas or comments, or just answer a question inappropriately. He doesn't notice that his behavior is disconcerting to others. Memory lapses may become increasingly common. A developing drinking problem may prompt trouble at work, such as failure to carry out responsibilities that used to be done reliably. The drinker may lose interest in hobbies and outside events in general. In addition, he may stop caring about his appearance and the appearance of his home, garden, car, or whatever else was previously important to him.

2. Changes in drinking patterns. Switching from beer to liquor, drinking at home when that wasn't a habit before, and going out more often to drink are all changes in drinking patterns that may indicate a problem with alcohol. If your partner begins to lie about his drinking (to say he has been working late when he has been at a bar, for example), or begins to disappear frequently for short intervals, he may have a drinking problem.

3. Changes in physical health. Signs to watch out for include easy bruising (caused by vitamin deficiencies), increasingly frequent bouts of ill health, morning vomiting, lack of physical coordination, and lack of appetite. Changes in mental health might include anxiety, depression, and insomnia.

Defining Alcoholism

"He has a drinking problem." No doubt you've heard this phrase before and may have used it yourself to describe someone who drinks more than is considered socially acceptable in most communities. What's the difference between a drinking problem and alcoholism? Addiction. An alcoholic is a person who would go through withdrawal if he stopped drinking alcohol. A problem drinker, on the other hand, would not. Although a problem drinker isn't addicted, he or she frequently gets into trouble when drinking. That trouble might be anything from getting drunk and sick, to engaging in abusive behavior, to driving while intoxicated (thus endangering the lives of others as well as their own). Thus both types of drinkers are likely to have family, social, health, work, financial, and legal problems as a result of their drinking.

The American Medical Association defines alcoholism as a chronic disease that develops from a combination of genetic, psychological, social, and environmental factors. The disease often gets worse over time and can be fatal. In fact, alcohol abuse kills about 100,000 Americans per year. That's more than six times the number who die from the use of all the illegal drugs—such as cocaine and heroin—put together.

Typically, alcoholics can't control their drinking, are preoccupied with drinking, and continue to use alcohol despite negative consequences. Many deny that they have a drinking problem.

For those who are physically addicted to alcohol, quitting is very difficult and staying sober is a lifelong challenge. "Five years into our marriage, my husband, Sam, almost died from alcoholism," says Marie (names have been changed to protect privacy). "He ended up in the hospital not knowing if he would make it physically or mentally. Within a month, he walked out and, from that time on, he never touched alcohol."

While Sam was in the hospital, he was introduced to programs and resources in the community designed to help alcoholics. He and Marie learned that alcoholism is a disease, not a personal weakness or anyone's fault. "I learned that I didn't cause Sam's alcoholism, and I can't cure it," says Marie. "There were other alcoholics in the hospital with Sam who blamed their drinking on their wives or on problems at work. But Sam said: 'They don't know what's wrong with them, but I do.' " From then on Sam went to meetings of Alcoholics Anonymous, which defines itself as "a fellowship of men and women who share their experience, strength, and hope with each other that they may solve their common problem and help others to recover from alcoholism." The only requirement for membership is a desire to stop drinking.

 ARE YOU TROUBLED BY SOMEONE'S DRINKING?
This questionnaire was created by Al-Anon, an international support organization for those whose lives have been adversely affected by someone else's drinking problem. If you answer Yes to three or more of these questions, Al-Anon may be able to help you. Check your phone book for a local Al-Anon group, or call 1–800–344–2666 for a meeting near you. Al-Anon also has a Web site at www.al-anon.org/.

1. Do you worry about how much someone else drinks?
2. Do you have money problems because of someone else's drinking?
3. Do you tell lies to cover up for someone else's drinking?
4. Do you feel that if the drinker loved you, he or she would stop drinking to please you?
5. Do you blame the drinker's behavior on his or her companions?
6. Are plans frequently upset or canceled or meals delayed because of the drinker?
7. Do you make threats, such as: "If you don't stop drinking, I'll leave you"?
8. Do you secretly try to smell the drinker's breath?
9. Are you afraid to upset someone for fear it will set off a drinking bout?
10. Have you been hurt or embarrassed by a drinker's behavior?
11. Are holidays and gatherings spoiled because of drinking?
12. Have you considered calling the police for help in fear of abuse?
13. Do you search for hidden alcohol?
14. Do you often ride in a car with a driver who has been drinking?
15. Have you refused social invitations out of fear or anxiety?

16. Do you sometimes feel like a failure when you think of the lengths to which you have gone to control the drinker?
17. Do you think that if the drinker stopped drinking, your other problems would be solved?
18. Do you ever threaten to hurt yourself to scare the drinker?
19. Do you feel angry, confused, or depressed most of the time?
20. Do you feel there is no one who understands your problems?

Get the Help *You* Need

Marie had already started attending local meetings of Al-Anon, an organization that offers "a self-help recovery program for the families and friends of alcoholics—whether or not the alcoholic seeks help or even recognizes the existence of a drinking problem."

"Al-Anon saved my life," says Marie, who has been a member now for 40 years. "Sam's drinking had erased my identity as well as his own. I had forgotten how to laugh and didn't even realize it. When you love someone, it's very difficult to watch him destroying himself and his marriage. I gave well-meaning, good advice and tried to help in anyway I could think of. But it was never enough. Through Al-Anon, I learned that you have to let go and get on with your own life."

Once Marie understood and accepted that beating alcoholism was something Sam had to do himself and that his drinking wasn't a reflection on her, she was able to distance herself from the problem. "I had two little girls at the time," she says, "and I thought: 'Unless Sam gets healthy, they're not going to have two parents, but at least they *are* going to have one.' "

Marie went to work full-time to build a life that didn't rely on Sam, who drifted in and out of jobs. Marie loved her work, and realized that she could take care of her children alone if she had to. After two years, however, she decided that her working was making it easier for Sam to avoid his responsibility to his family. She quit her job to stay home with her children, one of whom had been born with Down syndrome.

"It was quite a roller-coaster ride until Sam became sober," she says. "And even then, we didn't find ourselves living in Utopia just because he stopped drinking. Relationship issues came up that had never come up before because alcoholism takes over everything. We had to work a lot of things out, but Sam is now 36 years sober and we recently celebrated our 45th wedding anniversary."

Most people who are alcohol-dependent need outside help, either from a program like Alcoholics Anonymous, from medical professionals, or both. However, as noted above, a woman can help by making sure her partner knows about community resources that are available to help alcoholics, and by getting counseling herself.

 HELP HOTLINES
  - American Council on Alcoholism: 1–800–527–5344
  - Alcoholism Hotline: 1–800–322–5525
- National Council on Alcoholism and Drug Dependence: 1–800–622–2255
- Domestic Violence Hotline: 1–800–799–SAFE
- National Child Abuse Hotline: 1–800–422–4453
- Al-Anon: 1–800–344–2666
- Alcoholics Anonymous: Look for a local AA phone number in your telephone directory.

Talk about Alcohol

Women whose partners have a drinking problem but aren't addicted can be supportive in additional ways. Rather than confronting a partner who drinks more than is considered healthy, therapists suggest encouraging him to talk about why he drinks and why he does or doesn't think his drinking is a problem. Encouraging a drinker to compare the consequences of his drinking to what he values in life may make him realize that the former is leading him away from the latter. That realization may be enough to mobilize his motivation to cut back.

For example, a woman might ask her partner how he feels the day after having three glasses of wine with dinner. Probably tired, not quite at the top of his game, maybe a little down. Often, the after-work-cocktail and wine-with-dinner habits are ones that aren't given much thought. Increasing a partner's awareness of the connection between the wine he drank at night and the way he feels—physically and mentally—the next day may make him think twice before drinking as much in the evening.

If you drink, too, cutting back with your partner is an important way that you can support his efforts. Before you both get started, each of you should keep a drink journal for a week, noting every drink you have, as well as the time of day and place or situation in which you have it. This will give you a good idea of whether you're drinking too much, and what situations you might want to avoid to make it easier to cut back. When formulating your plan, bear in mind that drinking with meals is better than drinking without food, and that drinking one or two beers daily is better than bingeing on six beers two times a week.

Discuss with your partner how drinking affects each of you and your relationship. For example, a couple of beers may relax a person enough that he or she feels comfortable sharing thoughts and feelings that might not otherwise be expressed. On the other hand, a few drinks makes some people more aggressive. Sexually speaking, alcohol has a mixed bag of effects. Generally, experts say, it increases the desire but diminishes the performance. A drink or two may lower each partner's inhibitions, making sex more exciting. However, too many drinks can inhibit erection, making sex quite dull. In nonmonogamous relationships, drinking reduces the odds that a condom will be used, which increases the risk of sexually transmitted disease. In any couple, alcohol may trigger arguments that wouldn't otherwise occur.

DEFINING MODERATION AND EXCESS

Experts recommend drinking "in moderation." In a society where one person's moderation is another person's excess, how do we know what level of drinking is compatible with health? In its official Dietary Guidelines, the government recommends that women drink no more than seven drinks per week, and men no more than 14. The intended interpretation is one or two drinks per night—not two nights of binge drinking. Scientists also believe that drinking alcohol with meals is better for the body than drinking without food.

Because one person's drink may equal another person's sip, here's the official definition of how much fluid constitutes one drink. If the beverage is beer, 12 ounces equals one drink; if it's wine, 4 to 5 ounces equals one drink; and if it's liquor, 1.5 ounces of 80-proof liquor equals one drink.

Alcohol and Good Health: Do They Mix?

The answer to that question is: it depends. Most recovered alcoholics should completely refrain from drinking. So should men who have certain medical conditions such as diabetes, uncontrolled hypertension, liver disease, abnormal heart rhythms, peptic ulcers, or sleep apnea. Alcohol also should be avoided by men and women who are taking certain medications. But what about everyone else? Researchers have found that for those who have no medical reason to avoid alcohol, *moderate* drinking (one or two drinks per day) appears to yield some health benefits. Consider these findings:

• Men who drink modest amounts—one or two drinks a day—live longer than heavy drinkers and nondrinkers. How does alcohol protect health? No one knows for certain, but experts suspect that the increased life expectancy of moderate drinkers is related to alcohol's ability to help people manage stress.

• Resveratrol, a natural chemical that's plentiful in the skin of grapes, may offer protection from both cancer and high cholesterol. Red wine, which is made from whole grapes including the skin, is high in resveratrol. However, most experts believe that alcohol itself is what protects the heart. Resveratrol adds minimal additional benefits. So if your man prefers beer, white wine, or scotch, don't bother trying to convince him to switch.

• Heart-disease risk among people who consume one beer, one glass of wine, or one highball a day is 25 to 45 percent lower than it is among nondrinkers. In fact, experts estimate that alcohol prevents as many as 80,000 deaths from heart disease each year in the U.S. However, *excessive* alcohol consumption *increases* a person's risk of heart disease.

• In an 11-year study of more than 22,000 male physicians aged 40 and older, researchers found that those who drank two to six alcoholic drinks a week were 21 to 28 percent less likely to die during the study than men who had just one drink per week. However, they also found that men who drank two or more drinks a day increased their risk of death by 50 percent.

• Drinking beer may help to prevent kidney stones. Researchers in Seattle found that men who drink beer are 53 percent less likely to form kidney or bladder stones than men who don't. In the study, one 8-ounce glass a week was enough to reduce the risk.

On the other hand . . .

• Alcohol is associated with about 100,000 deaths from diseases and injuries in the U.S. each year.

• Alcohol has been linked to several types of cancer, including lung, esophageal, gastric, pancreatic, and urinary tract.

• Compared to moderate drinkers and nondrinkers, people who abuse alcohol have double the risk of death from homicide or suicide.

• Heavy drinkers suffer brain shrinkage (loss of brain cells), and even moderate drinking may affect brain function.

• Heavy drinking can cause fatty deposits in the liver, eventually leading to cirrhosis. A liver damaged by alcohol cannot process the nutrients in food nor eliminate toxins from the blood.

• Alcohol is a common cause of gastritis and stomach bleeding.

• Alcohol is an important cause of hypertension, which is a cause of stroke.

• Despite initially helping to relieve tension, alcohol can actually heighten anxiety. It's also a factor in many cases of depression.

• Taken often and in large quantities, alcohol is addictive.

• Excessive alcohol consumption has been linked to various other personal health problems, including vitamin deficiency, obesity, sexual dysfunction, infertility, muscle disease, skin problems, and pancreatitis.

• Excessive alcohol use is associated with more than half of all violent deaths in the United States (causes range from murder to drowning to death by fire).

No expert would suggest that a nondrinker start drinking for the health benefits. However, as mentioned above, healthy men who already drink occasionally won't do their health any harm. The key is moderation, as the following statistic shows: middle-aged men who binge on beer—drinking six or more bottles at a time—have a six times greater risk of fatal heart attack, a seven times greater risk of dying violently, and a three times greater risk of dying overall compared with men who drink less than three bottles per session.

Herman Johannsen, the cross-country skier who lived to be 111, put it nicely when he offered this advice to those seeking longevity: "Stay busy, get plenty of exercise, and don't drink too much. Then again, don't drink too little, either."

Take an honest look at how alcohol is affecting your lives and your relationship. Only then will you be in a position to make better choices about how often and how much to drink. Remember, alcohol is like a spice: it tastes good and complements the dish of life, but too much can ruin your meal.

 THIRTEEN WAYS TO HELP YOUR MAN CUT BACK
Here are 13 ways you and your man can reduce alcohol consumption over a period of time, courtesy of the British agency Alcohol Concern:

1. Go out a bit later than you usually do, or go out at your usual time but have your first drink later in the evening.

2. Replace some of your drinks with nonalcoholic beverages. Make every other drink a glass of water, juice, or soda.

3. Switch your usual drink to one with less alcohol in it. For example, drink beer or wine instead of mixed drinks.

4. Avoid "quick drinks." Don't have a drink while you're getting dressed to go out, skip alcohol at lunch, and don't grab a "quick drink" before heading home after work. These small changes can make a huge difference over the course of a week.

5. Drink longer drinks. In other words, choose something you sip over something you shoot.

6. Decide on a limit of, say, no more than four drinks on any one occasion.

7. If you anticipate a heavy evening, avoid drinking on an empty stomach and make sure someone else is driving.

8. Tell others you're cutting down and avoid participating in the buying of rounds.

9. Have at least two alcohol-free days per week. If you find that most of your social life centers around drinking, take up a new interest or sport, or just go to the movies more often.

10. If you drink at home, buy beers and wines with lower alcohol contents—it could make a great difference.

11. Buy smaller glasses for the home or buy a shot measure so that drinks you make yourself won't be larger than a standard-sized drink.

12. Keep a supply of tasty nonalcoholic alternatives at home for your own use and for entertaining.

13. Find other ways of relaxing. Try exercise or relaxation techniques, for example. Head for the bedroom instead of the bar.

9

GIVE STRESS THE SLIP

By the age of 37, Danny Shainis had had two heart attacks. His doctors identified stress as one of the risk factors he needed to control. "When Danny's under pressure, his arteries start to spasm," says his wife, Marcia. "Prior to his first heart attack, he also smoked and had high cholesterol, so he had a few factors working against him."

Danny quit smoking after his first heart attack, and with Marcia's help, began following a low-fat, low-cholesterol diet (see Chapter 4, "Create a Healthy Kitchen," to find out how the couple changed their eating habits). But what about stress? A man in his early forties, Danny's in the midst of a successful career in apparel sales. He commutes to New York City from Connecticut daily during the week, except when he's out of town on business. Add to that a young daughter, a working wife, and a large network of family and friends with whom the couple wants to stay in touch, and you've got the makings for a big bowl of stress soup.

After Danny's second heart attack, he and Marcia took

several steps to slow down the pace of their lives. To help him learn new ways of dealing with work-related stress, Danny started seeing a psychotherapist. Through therapy, he also came to understand patterns in his behavior that increased the demands of his personal life, making it a source of stress, too. For example, he tended to internalize other people's problems, taking them on as if they were his own. "Our biggest challenge," says Marcia, "was to start saying No to friends more often. Danny has now learned to plan his free time better, focusing on what's important to him rather than overextending himself socially. He's still there for his friends, but we don't do weekends jam-packed with social events any more. We're much more realistic about our time and energy limitations."

Recently, the Shainises took their stress-reduction campaign to the next level. They reevaluated their lives from several perspectives: personal, professional, physical, and financial. "We looked around our big house and decided that the three of us didn't need all that space and all those things," says Marcia. "We sold a lot of stuff, including our house, and moved into a three-bedroom cluster home. The more things you get rid of, the less stress you have. There's just less to worry about."

Choosing to rent instead of own has eliminated many hassles. When something goes wrong with the plumbing or with an appliance, Marcia makes a call and it gets fixed at no cost to the Shainises. They don't have to maintain a yard or shovel a driveway.

Although the couple has made major changes to reduce anxiety on the home front, Danny's work remains a major source of stress. He has episodes of angina (chest pain caused by a temporary shortage of the supply of blood to the heart), almost all of which occur at work when he's under pressure.

Although the step would be a drastic one, changing jobs might be the best way for Danny to manage his work-related stress and potentially prolong his life significantly. "It's not easy for a man in his forties at the height of his career to walk away from it all," says Marcia. "Nevertheless, when you've already had three angioplasties, you want to make the right decisions."

Stress and Health

Stress is defined as "a physical, chemical or emotional factor that causes bodily or mental tension." It can prompt an astounding array of physical symptoms, from the cosmetic, like baldness, to the deadly, like heart attack. (See "How Stress Can Play Havoc With Your Body" on page 241 for a list of conditions that are linked to stress.)

Just what does stress do to cause so much trouble? When a person encounters a stressful situation, his or her body routinely responds by releasing various chemicals to prepare the body to fight or take flight. The adrenal glands release adrenaline and other hormones that cause the heart rate and blood pressure to increase. In addition, muscles tense for action, blood sugars and fat are released into the bloodstream for extra energy, and in case of injury, chemicals that make it easier for blood to clot are released. Pupils dilate so you can see better, perspiration increases to cool your body, and breathing accelerates to increase the amount of oxygen available in the blood.

Obviously, the appearance of stress and the usual bodily reaction to it can serve a person well under certain conditions. For example, it might boost mental performance in a job interview, increase stamina when a deadline is looming, or give you the strength to carry someone out of a burning house.

However, when a body spends lots of time in this hyper-alert state, it pays a price. Ongoing, unmanaged stress can depress the immune system's ability to fight disease, and increase risk of heart attack and stroke.

Stress affects the heart in several ways: it causes blood vessels to constrict, which increases blood pressure; it causes platelets to become stickier than they should be, which makes clots more likely; and it cuts testosterone levels, which reduces "good" cholesterol and increases triglycerides (a type of blood fat that's linked to heart disease).

Duke researchers divided a group of 107 adults with coronary disease and ischemia into three subgroups. The first received standard medical care only; the second received exercise training; the third received weekly therapy sessions during which they learned about the links between psychosocial stress and heart disease. These patients were also taught how to reduce stress through relaxation and biofeedback techniques. Five years after the study, those people who underwent four months of stress-management training had only a 9 percent incidence of cardiac events (defined as heart surgery, angioplasty, heart attack, or death), compared to 30 percent of patients who received standard medical care. Patients in the exercise group had a lower relative risk for cardiac events than did patients in the group that received medical care only, but the effect wasn't statistically significant.

HOW STRESS CAN PLAY HAVOC WITH YOUR BODY

Prolonged stress has been linked to the following conditions:

- Angina
  (pain in the chest caused by a temporarily inadequate supply of blood to the heart)
- Anxiety
- Baldness
- Behavioral and emotional problems
- Bruxism (grinding of teeth)
- Canker sores
- Chronic fatigue
- Cold sores
- Depression
- Dyspepsia
  (stomach cramps and discomfort not linked to a specific cause)
- Skin disorders, including eczema, dermatitis, psoriasis, hives, and acne
- Headache
- Heart attack
- High blood pressure
- Impotence
- Indigestion
- Insomnia
- Irritable bladder
- Irritable bowel
- Menstrual disorders
- Migraine
- Muscle aches
- Muscle twitches and tics
- Obesity
- Premature ejaculation

Work: The Most Common Stressor

Researchers looking into what causes negative stress responses have made some observations that might help you and your partner isolate the causes of ongoing stress in your lives. One of the biggest work-related stressors that can make for trouble is lack of control over workplace decisions. A British study of more than 7,000 civil servants between the ages of 35 and 55 found that, compared with those at the top of the bureaucratic ladder (administrators), clerical and office-support staff displayed an approximately 50 percent increased risk for heart disease.

Interestingly, the researchers concluded that work demands themselves don't increase a person's risk for heart disease. Rather, the issue appears to be how much control he or she has over work-related issues.

Another study, this one done in Finland, followed nearly 1,000 middle-aged men for four years. Researchers found that low income was a risk factor for carotid atherosclerosis (hardening of the arteries), a condition that increases risk of heart attack and stroke.

The message these studies send—ditch that low-control job and try to earn more money—isn't as impractical as it may seem. For example, someone working as one of 50 accountants in a big company may find more job control and satisfaction working as one of two accountants in a small firm. Employees in small firms are much more likely to have input into company policy and decision-making than those in large companies, which tend to have clear-cut chains of command and less flexible systems.

If your partner isn't earning as much as he'd like to, help him realize that he does have options. Additional schooling or vocational training may help him step up his earnings over time. Perhaps he'd be better off in a different, more lucrative field. In some cases, it may even pay off in the long run to take a step down in income in exchange for training in an area where earning potential is higher.

Having a specific goal and working toward that goal will help to relieve the frustrations of a low-control job. For example, a man who works as a gas-station attendant might ask the station owner what he would need to accomplish in order to be promoted to a manager. His ultimate goal might be to own his own station. As the legendary Chinese philosopher Lao-tzu said: "The journey of a thousand miles begins with a single step."

Change is another common sources of stress. Positive changes, such as getting married or having a child, can be as stressful as negative changes, such as divorce or the death of a loved one. Experts agree that stress doesn't become a problem until the demands outweigh one's personal resources for dealing with them positively. That may occur when several stressors that would have been manageable on their own converge in a person's life. Or it could happen when one usually intermittent and manageable stressor becomes an ongoing problem. Naturally, some individuals can tolerate more stress than others.

WHY SLEEP IS IMPORTANT—AND HOW TO GET MORE

Stress is a common cause of insomnia, but as with the chicken and the egg, it can be difficult to determine which came first: the stress or the sleeplessness? With every passing year, it seems that people find more reasons to stay up longer and not "waste" time sleeping. Working parents try to cram time with their children into the hours after dinner, often resulting in later bedtimes for the children. That, in turn, may prompt the parents to stay up a little longer—after all, nighttime is the only time they have to themselves all day. One can grocery-shop, cruise the Internet, or watch television 24 hours a day in most places. And of course, there are always bills to pay, books to read, and friends and family with whom to keep in touch.

Although some people say they feel fine on less than the recommended eight hours of sleep each night, chronic sleep deprivation can accumulate and cause physical problems such as depression and anxiety. An ongoing sleep deficit also can reduce a person's energy level and impede his or her ability to think clearly and logically.

What can you and your partner do to make sure you get enough sleep? The first step is to set a bedtime and do your best to stick to it. If you have to get up at 6 A.M. every weekday morning, you know you should aim to be in bed with the lights out at 10 P.M. Work backwards from there to calculate the times at which your evening activities will have to take place in order for you to meet that goal. For example, if you want two hours to yourselves each night, you know that dinner will have to be over, the dishes done, and the children tucked in by 8 P.M. If it takes 45 minutes to get the children into their pajamas, teeth brushed, stories read, and songs sung, you'll have to start that process at 7:15 P.M. every night. That may mean the kids have to be in the bath tub by 6:45 P.M., and dinner has to be served at 6 P.M.

If you and your partner don't have children, your schedule can be less regimented. However, you should still plan to have dinner at the same time every night, say 7 P.M., so that you'll have your downtime and still can be abed by 10! If you don't usually crawl between the sheets until 11 or 12 P.M., move your bedtime back gradually. Try half-hour increments.

If you're having trouble sleeping, there are several things you can try to make it easier for the sandman to do his job:

• **Schedule workouts to maximize sleep.** Don't exercise after 6 P.M. In the hours immediately following a workout, the body is extra alert, which can make it difficult to fall asleep. However, after four or five hours the body becomes very relaxed. So do take a brisk walk at 4:30 P.M. or 5 P.M.

- **Don't take naps during the day.** That can disrupt your sleep cycle and make it difficult to fall into the deep, restorative sleep you need at night.
- **Don't read in bed, unless it's a relaxing novel.** Books on serious subjects can set your mind spinning and make it difficult to turn your thoughts off with the lights.
- **Take a bath one or two hours before bedtime.** The warmth will wash away your worries.
- **Come up with one or two relaxing fantasies to help you fall asleep.** Conjure up images of a cozy bed in a cabin in the woods or a lounge chair on the beach. Imagine that you're falling asleep there without a care in the world.
- **Try not to bring up important family issues in bed.** Sometimes it seems that bedtime is the only time a couple has to communicate all day, but you'll have trouble relaxing after discussing your teenage daughter's newly pierced nose.
- **Don't drink more than a cup or two of caffeinated drinks during the day.** Avoid them altogether after dinner. Warm milk with honey and certain herb teas may help you relax and make it easier to fall asleep.
- **Avoid drinking a lot of alcoholic beverages.** A drink may initially make you sleepy, but even moderate amounts of alcohol can disrupt normal sleep patterns.
- **Make time to talk with your partner.** Sit down after dinner and help each other come up with ways to solve problems and fit errands into the family schedule. If your partner is having trouble with a coworker, help him come up with a course of action. If you have several errands to run in the week before your son's birthday party, divide up the work and plan when each thing can be accomplished. Laying out what you need to do and seeing that it can all be accomplished will leave you both free to relax and slumber peacefully.

Symptoms of Stress Overload

According to the American Medical Association and other authorities, signs of excess or unmanageable stress include difficulty sleeping; significant weight gain or loss; social withdrawal or frantic social activity; working a lot more or a lot less than usual; behaving in a more tense or emotional manner than usual; drinking or smoking more than usual; constant headaches or muscular pains not otherwise explainable; change in bowel or urinary habits; the appearance of hives or certain other skin disturbances; and the occurrence of muscular tics.

Be especially vigilant if your partner is in the midst of any of the situations listed below because they put him at increased risk for stress-related illness.

- Death of a loved one
- Job loss or retirement
- Divorce or separation
- Decreased income
- Loan or mortgage foreclosure
- Marital separation
- Major change in health or behavior of a family member
- Marriage or reconciliation after a separation
- Hospitalization—his own or that of a loved one
- Major dental work
- Problems at work, especially loss of control
- Taking on substantial debt such as a mortgage
- Changing jobs
- Problems at school

Anger: A Dangerous Response to Stress

Do hassles and inconveniences make your man tense up like a cobra ready to strike? Does he step on the gas instead of the brake when he sees a yellow warning light? Does he get angry when faced with everyday inconveniences like waiting on line or driving behind someone who thinks turn signals are for decoration? If so, your partner may be at increased risk for a heart attack.

People react to negative stress in various ways. Some become overwhelmed, anxious, or even depressed; others become hostile. Anxiety and depression can be treated, but hostility isn't considered a condition that calls for medical intervention. However, in view of current research, one could argue that hostility is a risk factor for heart disease— just like smoking or eating a high-fat diet—and it should be treated as such.

In his best-selling book, *Anger Kills,* Dr. Redford Williams warns that people who have an angry response to everyday setbacks—most of whom are men—are four to seven times more likely to be dead of coronary disease and other causes by age 50 than those who are more tolerant of minor annoyances. Each time a person has a hostile reaction to a situation, fat is released into the bloodstream to provide energy for the fight—or flight—the body thinks might lie ahead. When neither occurs, the fat remains in the blood where it can collect as plaque on artery walls. As explained in Chapter 3, "Boost Your Nutrition Knowledge," plaque increases the odds that a heart attack or stroke will occur.

What can you do if your partner is quick to anger in everyday situations? Williams and other experts recommend exercise. It helps burn off the extra fat—and the mental steam. In addition to encouraging him to exercise (see Chapter 5, "Get Your Man Moving," for how-tos), you can help your man become more aware of his irate reactions to common situations such as getting stuck in traffic, and of how that anger can harm his health.

Encourage your man to look at each situation in a larger context. Yes, it's annoying when someone doesn't signal a turn, but is it something that should spoil your whole morning? Learning to let go of things over which he has no control, such as other people's actions and behavior, will significantly reduce your partner's hostility. Next time your man finds himself held up in line at the post office, suggest that he use the time to people watch, think about what he wants to do over the weekend, read the newspaper, or come up with a special gift he can buy for your next birthday.

CHECK OUT THESE INTERNET STRESS SITES

For more information about stress and its effects, or to connect with others who feel under the gun, surf to these useful Web sites:

- **Biobehavioral Institute of Boston:** http://www.bbinst.org/home2. html. This site offers information on stress, its effects, and its management. There's an interactive forum and a "stress audit" designed to evaluate the pressures in your life.
- **Virtual Psyche:** http://www.geocities.com/~virtualpsych/. Another good site that includes useful information about stress and its management. This one is written by a clinical psychologist. Look here if you want to know more about cognitive therapy (changing the way you look at things) and other long-term stress-management techniques. The site also includes interesting stress facts, relaxation techniques, and tips on how to build better relationships.
- **The Web's Stress Management and Emotional Wellness Page:** http://imt.net/~randolfi/StressPage.html. In addition to a discussion forum and inspiring quotations relating to stress and emotional health, this site provides lots of helpful links divided into categories. These include cognitive ap-

proaches, relaxation techniques, stress in the workplace, chronic arousal interventions, and situational interventions.

Prune Excess Stress

Now what? You understand that stress can damage health, and you've discussed the issue with your partner. But what can you do about it? You can't quit your jobs, pack the children off to Grandma's and spend your days meditating, preparing healthy meals, and letting the answering machine pick up the phone.

Even if you could avoid all the people, places, and events that sometimes make your lives stressful, chances are you wouldn't want to. Life without challenges would be boring indeed. Instead, your goal should be to avoid stressful situations that don't serve some purpose in your lives, and to effectively manage the stress that you can't—or don't want to—avoid.

In a relationship, if one partner manages stress poorly, the other will no doubt be affected directly. Often, in fact, he or she becomes a "safe target," someone on whom the stressed-out partner can vent his or her frustrations and anxiety. Think about it: most of us try to avoid arguing with coworkers, neighbors, and people waiting in line at the grocery store. On the other hand, most of us expect to argue with our partners. We understand that it would be virtually impossible to share our lives with another person without disagreeing about issues large and small on a fairly regular basis. That's why it's vital to work together to manage stress in positive ways.

Stress is a sly thief, frequently snatching health and peace of mind from people without their realizing they've been robbed. Most people attribute symptoms such as frequent colds, muscle aches, and fatigue to bad luck or advancing age. They're reluctant to admit that physical ills could be rooted in a psychological cause, such as unmanaged or poorly managed stress. That's a shame, because it's impossible to defeat an enemy you don't acknowledge.

In Marcia Shainis's opinion, stress reduction is a top priority for couples who want to live healthier lives. For those who groan at the thought of adding time for stress management to their daily routine, Marcia suggests stealing time from meal preparation. "Take time to cut back the clutter in your lives and find ways to reduce the demands that you place on yourselves. After all, you only eat three times a day, and there are plenty of healthy foods that require little preparation. Stress, however, is a continuous challenge."

FIFTEEN WAYS YOU AND YOUR PARTNER CAN FIGHT STRESS

The list below contains ideas that will help you and your partner eliminate some pressures and better manage the others:

1. Avoid negative thinking. Pay attention to your "self-talk" (the thoughts that run through your mind). Is it positive or negative? Here's an example of positive self-talk: "I missed the promotion this time, but I'll talk to my boss and find out which areas I need to improve in so that I won't be passed over next time."

A negative response to the same situation might go something like this: "I didn't get the promotion because my work isn't good enough. I'll be in this same job forever." Or: "I'm good enough, but my boss and just about every one else above me is prejudiced against me. I'll never get ahead, no matter how hard I try. I'm just a victim." Words like "always," "forever," "every time," and "never" are tip-offs that thinking has turned negative.

Extreme words like these rarely paint an accurate picture of reality. If you catch yourself or your partner falling into this trap, try to respond with a positive interpretation of the situation in question. Learning not to overreact to situations will go a long way toward reducing stress.

2. Don't be a perfectionist. Perfectionists use the same type of all-or-nothing language as negative thinkers. "If it isn't perfect, it must be terrible." In reality, nothing is or can be perfect, so we shouldn't expect perfection from ourselves. Because perfectionism is an unattainable goal, it creates loads of negative stress.

Let's say your partner had a presentation at work and came home complaining that he forgot to discuss one whole section of the project, thus ruining his presentation. You have several response options. You could show empathy by saying: "Oh no, how awful." However, commiserating isn't going to make him feel any better or reduce his negative feelings. Instead, you might respond by helping him put his error in context. Ask whether anyone appeared to notice the exclusion, and how people responded to the rest of his presentation. To make up for the error, suggest that he consider circulating a memo to those who attended the meeting, summarizing the part of the presentation he left out.

3. Control your anger. As we pointed out earlier, people who get angry over the minor inconveniences and hassles of everyday life are at increased risk for heart attack and other stress-related illnesses. Of course, there are times when it's okay to feel anger. For instance, if you discover that someone you trust has gone back on his or her word. However, it's almost never helpful to let anger determine your actions.

When you feel anger coming on, ask yourself these three questions: Is this situation worth reacting to? Is my anger justified? Can I do anything to remedy the situation? If the answers are No, calm yourself down by putting the situation in perspective. For example, "My getting angry at the man who's tying up the checkout line arguing about coupons won't accomplish anything. In fact, the man might even feel bad about holding everyone up. Waiting patiently won't hurt me. In fact, I can put the time to good use by coming up with a way to improve relations with my restaurant's clientele."

4. Cut back on social engagements. Many of us feel we can't say No to an invitation unless we already have plans to go out on the night in question. Remind yourselves that it's okay to turn down an invitation for the simple reason that you'd like to spend some time alone with your partner, or because you've been so busy at work you just want to kick back and watch a video.

5. Remember that life is a journey, not a race. Avoid fast-food restaurants out of principle. Food isn't supposed to be fast, it's supposed to be good. And it's supposed to provide your body with the nutrients it needs to stay healthy. Don't do all your workouts in the gym. Yes, that may be the most efficient way to go—you can exercise your heart and every other muscle in your body all under one roof. But if you play tennis, hike, or go for a bike ride, your workout will be an experience instead of just another item on your to-do list. Picture someone writing the story of your life. Will it read like a richly detailed novel in which every day is of value, or like Crib Notes, in which only the highlights are worth mentioning?

6. Let go of guilt feelings and grudges. Both are big sources of stress that can be hard to get under control. If a decision you've made leaves you guilt-ridden, either rethink the decision or let go of the guilt and move on. The same goes for grudges. Either convince the person to right the wrong he did you, or forgive and forget. Far better to bury the hatchet than to allow the situation to continue to chip away at your peace of mind.

7. Don't rush. Try allowing yourselves 20 percent more time to accomplish a given task than your first instinct told you to allow. So if you estimate it will take you an hour to give the car a good cleaning, allow an hour and 12 minutes. This trick will help you to avoid rushing and being late, two common stressors.

8. Don't be afraid to take time off. We live in a fast-paced, work-oriented society. Many people behave as if they believe that you can tell all you need to know about someone by what they do for a living. The first question you're likely to be asked when meeting someone for the first time—even in a social setting—is: "What do you do?" Instead of saying: "I'm a sales representative" or "I drive a bus," wouldn't it be fun to surprise people with an answer like this: "I take photographs of wildlife, take my grandchildren on picnics, and play basketball whenever I get the chance." You can learn much more about who someone is by what they do on their own time than by what they do on someone else's.

Your time away from work is important. It's your chance to explore the range and depth of your talents and interests. Doing so will help you gain a larger respect for yourself and your abilities, and it will help you let go of everyday stress. However, this is one of those areas in life in which more isn't better. Trying to actively pursue several activities or interests will increase stress. Choose a couple of favorites, then relax and enjoy them.

9. Cut back on television. Watching television may appear to be relaxing—you just sit and stare. But studies have shown that some people feel less relaxed after watching television than they did before they sat down to watch. While we gaze at the tube, our brains are bombarded with visual and oral information. Your mind is ticking away trying to absorb all of this information and put it in context. This can be distracting rather than relaxing.

10. Get rid of some belongings. You may not realize it, but clutter is stressful. The more stuff you have around you, the more stuff you have to clean, organize, and fix when broken. One rule of thumb: if you haven't used it in a year, give it away, sell it, or throw it out.

11. Spend time alone. Our bodies respond to constant companionship by producing more stress hormones. We need time alone to let our minds wander, hash out ideas, and come to terms with events. You and your partner each should evaluate your needs and act accordingly. Some people can recharge on 20 minutes a day; others need more time to themselves.

12. Try relaxation exercises. Meditation, deep breathing, calming imagery exercises, biofeedback, and yoga all reduce stress. According to some experts, yoga carries an additional benefit—it improves sex by increasing a person's energy and flexibility. (Yoga postures that stretch tight muscles in the legs, hips, and pelvis are particularly beneficial for that purpose.)

13. Eat right. Stick to a diet that's low in fat and includes lots of fruits and vegetables, and not too much sugar, salt, alcohol or caffeine. (See Chapter 3, "Boost Your Nutrition Knowledge," for details.) In addition to all the other health benefits such a diet offers, it will provide your body with the resources it needs to manage stress successfully. Choosing a variety of healthy foods will help to ensure that you're getting enough of vitamins C, E, and B, which are thought to be of particular help to the body when it has psychological stress to handle.

14. Get moving. Going for a walk or playing softball may not seem very relaxing, but researchers have found that it is. In fact, when a group of students was divided into three groups, two that exercised and one that didn't, those who worked out for 20 minutes reduced their anxiety levels by 20 percent. Those who sat quietly in a room had the same level of anxiety after 20 minutes as they did before they sat down to relax.

15. Have sex frequently. Unfortunately, this may not be as easy as it sounds. Libido is one of the first things to head south when stress hits. Paradoxically, sex is one of the best destressors around. How can you and your partner overcome this hitch? Start by scheduling time to discuss problems at work or financial concerns before you tuck yourselves in. Such discussions make poor bedfellows. Then, head to bed half an hour earlier than usual. Don't think of this time as sex time, think of it as bonding time. Cuddle, hug, or give a massage. Talk about dreams of the future, endearing things the kids have said, or an upcoming vacation. You may or may not end up having intercourse on a given night, but the intimacy you create will in itself reduce stress. And odds are that sooner rather than later, you'll find yourselves eager to plunge into the ultimate act of intimacy.

10

BUILD A HEALTHY RELATIONSHIP

> *To fall in love is easy, even to remain in it is not difficult; our human loneliness is cause enough. But it is a hard quest worth making to find a comrade through whose steady presence one becomes steadily the person one desires to be.*
>
> *Anna Louise Strong*

Assuming that you've found your life comrade, how do you set about becoming—or remaining—a "steady presence," helping your man to become "the person [he] desires to be"? That's the fundamental question we've been indirectly addressing throughout this book. We've discussed the importance of educating your partner in a supportive manner about his health risks, setting a good example with your own behavior, and helping your partner make time for healthy habits, from exercise to meditation. In this chapter, we'll look specifically at how to build and maintain a healthy relationship—one strong enough to serve as a foundation from which both partners can become the people they want to be.

Although not commonly thought of as part of a health-maintenance program, good relationships are just that. Studies have shown that stable, happy relationships are protective against illness and premature death. Poor social relationships, on the other hand, are damaging to health—as damaging as cigarette smoking, some experts say. In a study done at Ohio State University, researchers asked 90 couples to discuss their most sensitive issues (the family finances, for example). Immune-system function and blood pressure were (the family finances, for example). Immune-system function and blood pressure were measured before and after the couples discussed their touchy topics. The results were that immune-system functioning dropped in all the participants, especially those displaying the most negative behaviors (accusing, criticizing, withdrawing). Those displaying negative behaviors also experienced a significant rise in blood pressure which lasted at least half an hour.

Good relationships help to foster health, but the opposite is also true: Healthy lifestyles help to foster good relationships. Since Roman LePree and his financée, Michelle Bromley, revamped their diets and started to exercise routinely, they've noticed an improvement in their relationship. "When you have a better image of yourself, it shows in your relationship," says Michelle. "You can be a lot more open with each other when you feel good about yourselves. We have a lot more fun than we used to."

SIGNS THAT A RELATIONSHIP IS IN TROUBLE

If the following behavior patterns fit your relationship, you and your partner might want to consider seeking professional counseling or signing up for a relationship-skills course (see "Resources for Better Relationships" on page 260):

- Habitual attempts to avoid each other
- Frequent arguments that don't get resolved
- Avoidance of or dissatisfaction with sex
- Mentions of divorce or breakup during arguments
- Disagreements over how to raise the children
- Physical abuse of a spouse and/or children

Do You Read Me?

The most important characteristic of a healthy relationship is frequent and clear communication. The first step toward establishing or maintaining good communication is easy— make time to talk. Given the hectic schedules with which many couples have saddled themselves, achieving this seemingly simple goal may be a challenge. A good beginning would be to sit down with your partner for at least half an hour each evening. This will provide you with the time you need to talk about household matters, such as upcoming medical or dental appointments, children's activities, and social commitments. Once that's done, you can check up on each other's emotional status on both the home and work fronts. How are you each feeling? Pressured? Content? Anxious? Angry? Excited? Happy? Challenged (positively or negatively)? Up? Down? Why are you each feeling the way you do?

Five simple house rules can help you create the time you need with your partner to keep the lines of communication open and static free.

1. Limit television watching. Certainly don't watch television during dinner. Beyond that, each family will have to make its own decisions about evening television watching. Just make sure that after fulfilling your obligations to any children or pets you may have, as well as personal obligations like exercise, you and your partner have time for your half-hour chat.

2. Limit telephone time. Don't make any phone calls after, say 9 P.M. unless absolutely necessary. This protects other people's downtime as well as your own. In addition, tell your friends and family to avoid calling after 9 P.M. One great way to limit phone calls is to use e-mail. If you have access to the Internet, e-mail allows you to communicate with others outside your household who also have Internet access about dates, times, plans and other factual information in an efficient and convenient manner. The sender and the receiver of the message can take part in the "conversation" at different times, depending on their personal schedules.

3. Limit evening errand running. If you and your partner tend to run out for everything from groceries to birthday cards and office supplies after dinner, try to limit your evening forays to once a week. If you can, go together. Then you can use the driving time for your nightly chat. Turn errand-running into an outing by stopping at a coffee house or an ice-cream parlor on your way home. If you can't go together, choose one night each and try to run all of your personal errands that night. Lumping three errands together is far more efficient than running out for one thing on each of three separate nights.

4. Exercise together. Working out with your partner allows you to kill two birds with one stone. You can talk to your partner and get fit, providing, of course, that the exercise you choose isn't so strenuous as to make talking difficult. Walking is perfect for couples who want to combine exercise with communication.

5. Try not to bring work home. Obviously, some jobs are easier to leave behind than others. A person whose job is dependent on equipment that remains at his or her place of work can't bring work home. But for many others, fax machines, computers, and cellular phones make it difficult not to. Nevertheless, regardless of how important a role someone plays at work, he or she has a more important obligation—to keep healthy. For most people, staying healthy means taking time for rest, exercise, and personal relationships.

Set Ground Rules for Talking

After you've created the time to talk, set some ground rules about how you'll discuss potentially volatile issues. Each partner should express any frustrations in terms of how the behavior in question affects him or her. For example, if your partner goes out for a beer or two after work three time a week, you might say: "When you're out after work, I feel lonely. I miss you and the children miss you. In addition, after caring for the children all day, I could use a break and some adult conversation. How would you feel about limiting your outings to once or twice a week, and occasional taking care of the children so that I can get out for a while with a friend?"

At the same time, it's essential to avoid personalizing the matter along "you're bad/I'm good" lines. If your partner resists your suggestion(s), try to keep the conversation feelings-focused, showing that you're aware he has them. Ask him why he feels he needs this time away from home, and why he doesn't feel you're entitled to the same. Try to find out why he feels he can't feed his children dinner and tuck them into bed unassisted. Of course, all of these questions must be asked out of a genuine desire to get to the bottom of this problem. Focus on the problem and solving it, not on the other person and his responsibility for it. Sarcasm will make it sound as if you're just blowing off steam or picking a fight, so avoid it at all costs.

When one partner is speaking, the other should listen quietly until that person is finished expressing his or her thoughts. Then the listening partner should paraphrase back what he or she has heard. If the listener has correctly understood the speaker, the listener should have a turn expressing his or her thoughts and feelings.

When a clear understanding of the problem has been reached and both partners have stated their needs and points of view, it's time for brainstorming. Work together to come up with a solution that both partners can live with. Doing nothing—in other words, leaving the situation as it is—shouldn't be considered an option. Unless the situation is at the "I don't love you anymore" level, it's almost always possible to come up with at least one mutually agreeable step that can be taken to help reduce one partner's dissatisfaction with a particular aspect of the relationship.

 RESOURCES FOR BETTER RELATIONSHIPS

The latest trend in the field of relationship reconstruction is classes designed to teach couples better strategies for airing grievances, resolving conflicts, and sustaining intimacy. Unlike traditional therapy for couples, this new breed of first aid for relationships has a straightforward goal—to improve participants' communication skills. The following programs are well established and widely available (for a more complete list of available programs, visit the Web site of the Coalition for Marriage, Family and Couples Education at http://www.smartmarriages.com):

- **PREP (Prevention and Relationship Enhancement Program).** This 12-hour class is offered at locations nationwide. For information on local classes, call 1–303–759–9931.

- **PAIRS (Practical Application of Intimate Relationship Skills).** This course is available in a variety of formats, from a one-day workshop to an intensive 120-hour program. For local classes, call 1–888–724–7748.
- **National Institute of Relationship Enhancement.** This group offers weekend workshops or coaching by phone, accessible from anywhere in the country. Call 1–800–432–6454.
- **Retrouvaille and Marriage Encounter.** Both programs are taught by trained couples rather than mental health professionals. The former is designed for deeply troubled marriages; the latter for stale relationships. Contact Retrouvaille at 1–800–470–2230; contact Marriage Encounter at 1–800–795–5683.

Building Blocks for Growth

If personal growth for both partners is to take place inside a relationship, two things are required: freedom and security—the freedom to experiment with change, and the security of knowing that someone is behind you regardless of whether you ultimately succeed or fail at making the change.

To enhance your partner's security, make sure he doesn't perceive that your love and respect for him are contingent upon his changing. It's easy to give this impression without realizing it. After all, simply suggesting a change in your partner's behavior implies that you're not satisfied with him as he is.

How can you get around this? First, spend some time considering exactly how you feel about whatever behavior it is that you'd like to see your partner change. Does his smoking make you angry? If so, why? Because it's harmful to your children's health? Because he shortens his life every time he lights up? Do you resent the expense of his smoking, or the way it makes your home smell? Do you find his smoker's breath unappealing? Next, think of ways to express your feelings without alienating your partner or making him feel that his place in your heart is in jeopardy. Instead, turn the discussion into an opportunity to reaffirm your love for him.

For example, you might say: "I love you and want you to be around for a long time because there are so many things I want us to do together in the future. Because smoking increases the odds that you'll die young, I would really like for you to try to quit smoking." Or, "I wonder if you realize that your smoking leaves a smell in the house that's really unpleasant for us nonsmokers. Together, let's try to come up with a solution to that problem."

Once you've expressed your feelings, ask about his. This is a step that's all too often forgotten. When no effort is made to solicit a partner's opinions and feelings, discussions about healthy habits tend to sound like marching orders: "This behavior isn't healthy, therefore you should change. I know what's best for you." That type of approach is almost certain to be perceived by a man as a threat to his personal freedom. Instead, show that you respect your man's independence by trying to draw out his feelings.

For example, try questions like these: "How do you feel about smoking? For you, what would be the hardest aspect of quitting? Do you want to quit? Why or why not? Would it be helpful if I took a walk with you every night after dinner? Would you like to avoid socializing with smokers for the first few weeks? Would you like me to make an appointment with your doctor so that you can discuss which smoking-cessation aid might be best for you?"

Asking what you can do to help is important because what you assume to be helpful may be highly annoying to your partner. For example, you may think that telling your partner's friends and family that he's going to quit smoking will establish a support network for him. He, on the other hand, may feel more secure quitting in private, so that he doesn't have to contend with the pressure of people constantly asking him how it's going.

Keeping your relationship strong is vital to the overall health of both you and your mate. In addition, without a solid and mutually satisfying partnership, it will be nearly impossible to help your man adopt healthier habits. So hunker down and get to work!

TEN WAYS TO NOURISH LOVE

In addition to offering your partner strong support and the freedom to grow and change, here are 10 more ways you can help to build a healthier relationship. Not only will you and your partner benefit, but your children will, too.

Offer unqualified support. Don't give your partner the impression that you'll love him more if he succeeds in changing and less if he doesn't. To thrive, a long-term relationship must be based on unqualified love.

1. Listen to each other. Countless marital disputes could probably be avoided if partners always allowed each other to complete their sentences. Too often, one partner assumes that he or she knows what the other intends to say. We're liable to attribute our own thoughts, fears, or insecurities to our partners, and before we know it an argument might be started over something that was never actually said. Couples can avoid this pitfall by following two well-proved rules of good communication, both of which it's particularly important to use during potentially volatile discussions: (1) allow each other to finish all sentences, and (2) always ask for clarification if you have any questions about what your partner is trying to say.

Because many men find it difficult to talk about their feelings, make sure you give your partner frequent opportunities to express himself in ways that are comfortable for him. Avoid the temptation to fill in any and all silences, so that he has a chance to formulate his thoughts and open up to you.

2. Focus on understanding each other, rather than on changing each other. Psychologists in Seattle compared two groups of patients who underwent marital counseling. One group received only traditional therapy, which teaches couples to avoid, or at least to prepare for, issues or situations that frequently spark disputes between them.

The other group received traditional therapy plus counseling designed to help them understand why their partners behaved in certain difficult ways. Wives and husbands had to try to see annoying acts as a result of personal history or psychological makeup. For example, a wife's temper might be an offshoot of her passionate involvement in life. A husband's difficulty expressing emotion might stem from the distant relationship that existed between his own parents. Rather, the goal was to inject enough tolerance and good will into each relationship to make partners want to change their destructive behavior.

After one year, eight of the nine couples who had tried the new approach said their relationships had improved substantially, and none had separated or divorced. Among the control group of 11 couples who received standard therapy, only half said their marriages had improved, and three of the couples had divorced or separated. The researchers concluded that accepting a partner—foibles and all—might be the ticket to moving beyond the stalemate that often surrounds recurring issues in a relationship. This was admittedly a small study; nevertheless, it makes an interesting point—the harder you try to change someone, the less likely he is to change.

3. Do nice things for each other on a daily basis. Showing that you care is just as important as saying so. If you're the first to leave for work in the morning, scrape the snow from his car windows when you do your own. Bring him a cup of tea or coffee if he's paying the bills. Most men will appreciate even the smallest gesture of tenderness and will most likely reciprocate with similar gestures toward you. Many people in relationships fall into the habit of concentrating on getting their own needs filled, whether social, psychological, practical, or sexual. Too often they think that the only way to get their partner to fulfill their emotional needs is to complain about current habits and ask for new ones. Worse, they don't say anything at all because they feel their needs are silly. Try showing your partner by example how you would like to be cared for. Once he understands from firsthand experience how wonderful it is to have a partner who routinely shows her love through small acts of kindness and consideration, he's almost certain to respond in kind.

4. Respect each other's pet peeves. If he can't stand it when you leave the cap off the toothpaste, get in the habit of putting it on when you're finished brushing. By the same token, he should remember to put the seat down after he uses the toilet. Why should either of you give in to requests that seem petty? Exactly because they are petty. Whereas you might not want to give in to your husband's wish that you home-school the children, why not humor him by remembering to note the date of an oil change in the car-maintenance file? Who knows? Maybe your efforts to accommodate your partner will prompt him to load silverware into the dishwasher with handles down (the way your mother always did) instead of up (the way his mother always did). The long and the short of it is that the more you and your partner can do to avoid irritating each other, the more fun it will be to live together.

5. Think of yourselves as a team. Too often partners become adversaries in a battle between his needs and her needs. Think of your relationship as a separate entity. Your goal should be to balance the needs of each individual with the needs of the partnership. Each partner must accept the fact that he or she will have to compromise in some situations and simply won't get what he or she wants in others. To foster the team spirit, focus on some long-term goals that you agree on. These goals could range from taking a trip to Europe or running a marathon together to sending one partner to school, saving for a house, starting a business, or having more time for your children. Decide how you'll reach each goal and work together to do so.

6. Have realistic expectations. If you don't, your partner will only disappoint you, and that feeling doesn't foster love. You may wish that your man still looked like he did when you met him, but no diet is healthy enough, nor any exercise regimen vigorous enough, to turn back the clock. Likewise, no amount of yoga or meditation can turn an adult with family responsibilities back into a carefree young man.

7. Do fun things together. Sounds simple, right? Yet how many of us manage to fit fun into daily schedules jammed with work, family, friends, fitness, cooking, cleaning, and laundry? For most couples, fun just isn't a priority. Nevertheless, if you can find a way to make time for it, you'll be well rewarded. Sheila Beahm and Larry Schulman have a love of outdoor activities in common. Together, they mountain-bike, hike, camp, rock climb, kayak, raft, and ski, among other things. "Being active is beneficial," says Larry, "and it's a lot more fun doing things with someone you care about." Sheila agrees: "Sharing all of these activities is a big part of the glue that holds us together."

Sheila and Larry are both established in their careers and have decided not to have children. That leaves them a lot of time for playing. Regardless of how much time you and your man can carve out for fun, your relationship will benefit from a shared hobby or activity.

8. Always speak with respect. If, in the heat of a given moment, you feel insults or other cruel words coming on, walk away. Excuse yourself, saying you need some time to cool off and think. Just remember that the partner who walks away from an argument bears the responsibility for returning and finishing the discussion when his or her thoughts are better formulated.

Avoid being accusatory or unnecessarily negative. That forces your partner to become defensive and increases the likelihood that he'll shut you out, which makes it virtually impossible to come up with a solution to the problem at hand.

9. Use humor carefully. Humor can help defuse tension—as long as your partner isn't the butt of a mean joke. Bear in mind that people vary in their ability to see the humor in their own behavior. If your partner can't laugh at himself, don't expect him to laugh when you tease him about his foibles, even if you're doing so in a good-natured way.

10. Last, but certainly not least, make love frequently. Physical love fosters emotional love in a way that's easy on the mind. It doesn't require putting feelings into words—something that most men aren't particularly enthusiastic about. Instead, it allows partners to connect on a level that goes beyond words to a place where souls can touch.

RESOURCES

Introduction
Why Should You Help Your Man Get Healthy?

Centers for Disease Control and Prevention. "Update: Prevalence of Overweight Among Children, Adolescents, and Adults—United States, 1988–1994." *Morbidity and Mortality Weekly Report* 46(9): 199–202, 1997.

Gurin, Joel. "The Us Generation." *American Health,* October 1985, pp. 40–41.

Kalish, Susan. *Your Child's Fitness: Practical Advice for Parents.* Champaign, Ill.: Human Kinetics, 1995.

"Lifestyles of the Old and Healthy: Predictors of Longevity in Men." *Harvard Men's Health Watch,* March 1997, pp. 6–7.

Manley, Audrey F. *Physical Activity and Health: A Report from the Surgeon General.* Washington, D.C.: U.S. Government Printing Office, July 1996.

Chapter 1
Mobilize Your Man's Motivation

Asnes, Marion. "Finding the Motivation." *Working Woman,* February 1994, pp. 56–61.

Gray, John. *Men Are from Mars, Women Are from Venus: A Practical Guide for Improving Communication and Getting What You Want in Your Relationships.* New York: HarperCollins, 1992.

Grilo, Carlos M. "The Power of Thinking in Weight Management." *The Weight Control Digest* 7(1): 585–591, 1997.

Jonas, Steven. "Regular Exercise: A Handbook for Clinical Practice," in *Motivation and Goal Setting.* New York: Springer, 1995.

———. *Take Control of Your Weight.* Yonkers, N.Y.: Consumer Reports Books, 1993.

Prochaska, James O., et al. "Working in Harmony with How People Change Naturally." *The Weight Control Digest* 3(3): 249–254, 1993.

Simon, Sidney B. *Getting Unstuck: Breaking Through Your Barriers to Change.* New York: Warner Books, 1988.

Tannen, Deborah. *You Just Don't Understand: Women and Men in Conversation.* New York: Ballantine Books, 1990.

Chapter 2
Share the Word on Screening

Bauman, Alisa, and Brian Kaufman. *Symptom Solver: Understanding—and Treating—the Most Common Male Health Concerns.* Emmaus, Penn.: Rodale Press, 1996.

Larson, David E., ed. *Mayo Clinic Family Health Book*. New York: William Morrow, 1996.

McGoon, Michael D., ed. *Mayo Clinic Heart Book*. New York: William Morrow, 1993.

Oppenheim, Michael. *The Men's Health Book*. Englewood Cliffs, N.J.: Prentice-Hall, 1994.

U.S. Department of Health and Human Services. *Prostate Cancer: Can We Reduce Mortality and Preserve Quality of Life?* Atlanta, Ga.: Centers for Disease Control and Prevention, 1997.

Chapter 3
Boost Your Nutrition Knowledge

American Heart Association. *1997 Heart and Stroke Statistical Update*. Dallas, Tex.: American Heart Association, 1997.

American Institute for Cancer Research. "Taking a Closer Look at Phytochemicals."

Appel, Lawrence J., et al. "A Clinical Trial of the Effects of Dietary Patterns on Blood Pressure." *New England Journal of Medicine* 336(16): 1117–1124, 1997.

Dietary Guidelines Advisory Committee. *Report of the Dietary Guidelines Advisory Committee on the Dietary Guidelines for Americans*. Washington, D.C.: U.S. Department of Agriculture, U.S. Department of Health and Human Services, 1995.

Gillman, Matthew W., et al. "Eating Fruits and Vegetables Lowers Risk of Stroke in Men." *Journal of the American Medical Association*, April 11, 1995.

Graham, I. M., et al. "Plasma Homocystein as a Risk Factor for Vascular Disease: The European Concerted Action Project." *Journal of the American Medical Association* 277: 1775–1781, 1997.

Herrmann, Howard C., ed. *Heart Watch: The 1997 Annual Heart Guide*. Waltham, Mass.: Massachusetts Medical Society, 1997.

McGoon, Michael D., ed. *Mayo Clinic Heart Book*. New York: William Morrow, 1993.

Moore, Thomas J. "Dietary Approaches to Stop Hypertension." *New England Journal of Medicine*, April 17, 1997.

Nestle, Marion, et al. "Guidelines of Diet, Nutrition, and Cancer Prevention: Reducing the Risk of Cancer with Healthy Food Choices and Physical Activity." *CA: A Cancer Journal for Clinicians* 46(6): 325–341, 1996.

Oppenheim, Michael. *The Men's Health Book*. Englewood Cliffs, N.J.: Prentice-Hall, 1994.

Perry, I. J., et al. "Prospective Study of Serum Total Homocysteine Concentration and Risk of Stroke in Middle-Aged British Men." *The Lancet* 346: 1395–1398, 1995.

Pyke, Stephen D., et al. "Change in Coronary Risk and Coronary Risk Factor Levels in Couples Following Lifestyle Intervention." *Archives of Family Medicine* 6: 354–360, 1997.

Rimm, Eric B., et al. "Vegetable, Fruit, and Cereal Fiber Intake and Risk of Coronary Heart Disease Among Men." *Journal of the American Medical Association* 275(6): 447–451, 1996.

Sifton, David W. *The PDR Family Guide to Nutrition and Health*. Montvale, N.J.: Medical Economics, 1995.

Wei, Ming, et al. "Total Cholesterol and High Density Lipoprotein Cholesterol as Important Predictors of Erectile Dysfunction." *American Journal of Epidemiology* 140(10): 930–937, 1994.

Chapter 4
Create a Healthy Kitchen

Blackburn, George. "Safe Amounts of Vitamins." *Health News,* August 26, 1997, p. 4.

Bredenberg, Jeff, and Alisa Bauman. *Food Smart: A Man's Plan to Fuel Up for Peak Performance*. Emmaus, Penn.: Rodale Press, 1996.

Dickey, Thomas, and Patricia A. Calvo, eds. *The Wellness Encyclopedia of Food and Nutrition*. New York: Rebus, 1992.

Hu, Frank. "Dietary Fat Intake and the Risk of Coronary Heart Disease in Women." *New England Journal of Medicine* 337: 1491–1499, 1997.

Liebman, Bonnie, and David Schardt. "Vitamin Smarts." *Nutrition Action Health Letter,* November 1995, pp. 6–10.

Sifton, David W. *The PDR Family Guide to Nutrition and Health*. Montvale, N.J.: Medical Economics, 1995.

Chapter 5
Get Your Man Moving

Blair, Steven N., et al. "Influences of Cardiorespiratory Fitness and Other Precursors on Cardiovascular Disease and All-Cause Mortality in Men and Women." *Journal of the American Medical Association* 276: 205–210, 1996.

Chichester, Brian, and Jack Croft. *Powerfully Fit: Dozens of Ways to Boost Strength, Increase Endurance, and Chisel Your Body*. Emmaus, Penn.: Rodale Press, 1996.

Klem, Mary I., et al. "A Descriptive Study of Individuals Successful at Long-Term Maintenance of Substantial Weight Loss." *American Journal of Clinical Nutrition* 66(2): 239–246, 1997.

Larson, David E., ed. *Mayo Clinic Family Health Book*. New York: William Morrow, 1996.

Williams, Paul T. "Relationship of Distance Run per Week to Coronary Heart Disease Risk Factors in 8283 Male Runners." *Archives of Internal Medicine* 157: 191–198, 1997.

Chapter 6
Protect Reproductive and Sexual Health

American Cancer Society. "Special Section: Prostate Cancer." *Cancer Facts and Figures,* 1998, pp. 20–24.

Appel, Lawrence, et al. "A Clinical Trial of the Effects of Dietary Patterns on Blood Pressure." *New England Journal of Medicine* 336(16): 1117–1124, 1997.

Berger, Richard. "New Name, New Treatments for Impotence." *HealthNews,* December 10, 1996, pp. 3–4.

Brawer, Michael K. "Treating Prostate Cancer." *HealthNews,* August 5, 1997, p. 3.

Food and Drug Administration. "FDA Approves Impotence Pill, Viagra." FDA Talk Paper, March 27, 1998.

Goldstein, Irwin, et al. "Oral Sildenafil in the Treatment of Erectile Dysfunction." *New England Journal of Medicine* 338(20): 1397–1404, 1998.

Simon, Harvey B., ed. "The Natural History of Benign Prostatic Hyperplasia." *Harvard Men's Health Watch* 2(8): 1–5, 1998.

Steinhauer, Jennifer. "Viagra's Other Side Effect: Upsets in Many a Marriage." *The New York Times,* June 23, 1998.

Chapter 7
Help Your Man Kick Butts

American Cancer Society. "Back Talk." From Web site http://www.cancer.org.

———. "Cancer Risk Report: Prevention and Control." 1996, pp. 1–4.

American Lung Association. "Nicotine Addiction and Cigarettes." From Web site http://www.lungusa.org.

———. "Protecting Yourself and Your Family from Secondhand Smoke."

Larson, David E., ed. *Mayo Clinic Family Health Book.* New York: William Morrow, 1996, pp. 315–324.

Nash, J. Madeline. "Addicted." *Time,* May 5, 1997, pp. 68–74.

"Passive Smoking: Even Worse Than We Thought." *UC Berkeley Wellness Letter,* January 1996, p. 2.

"Up in Smoke." *UC Berkeley Wellness Letter,* September 1997, p. 8.

Chapter 8
De-Emphasize Alcohol

"Alcohol: Weighing the Benefits and Risks for You." *UC Berkeley Wellness Letter,* August 1997, pp. 4–5.

Brody, Jane E. "Red Wine and Grapes May Inhibit Cancer." *The New York Times,* January 10, 1997.

"Healthy Limits for Alcohol." *HealthNews,* February 11, 1997, p. 6.

Larson, David E., ed. *Mayo Clinic Family Health Book.* New York: William Morrow, 1996, pp. 325–334.

Mason, Michael. "The Truth About Women and Wine." *Health,* May/June 1997, pp. 91– 98.

Chapter 9
Give Stress the Slip

American Medical Association. "The Effects of Stress," *AMA's Family Medical Guide CD-ROM.* New York: Dorling Kindersley Multimedia, 1997.

Gullette, Elizabeth C.D., et al. "Effects of Mental Stress on Myocardial Ischemia During Daily Life." *Journal of the American Medical Association* 277: 1521–1526, 1997.

Larson, David E., ed. *Mayo Clinic Family Health Book.* New York: William Morrow, 1996, pp. 307–314.

McGoon, Michael D., ed. *Mayo Clinic Heart Book.* New York: William Morrow, 1993, pp. 143–145, 172–177.

Chapter 10
Build a Healthy Relationship

Gray, John. *Men Are from Mars, Women Are from Venus: A Practical Guide for Improving Communication and Getting What You Want in Your Relationship.* New York: HarperCollins, 1992.

Levy, Ariel. "No Joy in Splitsville." *New York,* May 12, 1997.

Marano, Hara Estroff. "Rescuing Marriages Before They Begin." *The New York Times,* May 28, 1997.

"Marital Arguments Lead to Weakened Immune System in Older Couples." Ohio State University press release, March 12, 1996.

Tannen, Deborah. *You Just Don't Understand: Women and Men in Conversation.* New York: Ballantine Books, 1990.

INDEX